Report of Investigations 9674

Performance of a Polyurethane Core Seal Tested in a Hydrostatic Chamber

By Dennis R. Dolinar, Michael J. Sapko, and Samuel P. Harteis

DEPARTMENT OF HEALTH AND HUMAN SERVICES
Centers for Disease Control and Prevention
National Institute for Occupational Safety and Health
Pittsburgh Research Laboratory
Pittsburgh, PA

May 2008

Disclaimer

Mention of any company or product does not constitute endorsement by the National Institute for Occupational Safety and Health (NIOSH). In addition, citations to Web sites external to NIOSH do not constitute NIOSH endorsement of the sponsoring organizations or their programs or products. Furthermore, NIOSH is not responsible for the content of these Web sites.

Ordering Information

To receive documents or other information about occupational safety and health topics, contact NIOSH at

> Telephone: **1–800–CDC–INFO** (1–800–232–4636)
> TTY: 1–888–232–6348
> e-mail: cdcinfo@cdc.gov
>
> or visit the NIOSH Web site at **www.cdc.gov/niosh**.

For a monthly update on news at NIOSH, subscribe to NIOSH *eNews* by visiting **www.cdc.gov/niosh/eNews**.

DHHS (NIOSH) Publication No. 2008–129

May 2008

SAFER • HEALTHIER • PEOPLE™

CONTENTS

Page

ILLUSTRATIONS

CONTENTS—Continued

TABLES

ACRONYMS AND ABBREVIATIONS USED IN THIS REPORT

AASHTO American Association of State Highway and Transportation Officials
CFR   Code of Federal Regulations
LLEM   Lake Lynn Experimental Mine
LVDT   linear variable displacement transducer
MSHA   Mine Safety and Health Administration
NIOSH   National Institute for Occupational Safety and Health

UNIT OF MEASURE ABBREVIATIONS USED IN THIS REPORT

ft	foot
ft^2	square foot
ft^3/min	cubic foot per minute
g	gram
gal	gallon
gpm	gallon per minute
hp	horsepower
Hz	hertz
in	inch
in^3	cubic inch
lb	pound
lb/ft^3	pound per cubic foot
min	minute
psi	pound-force per square inch
sec	second
V/in	volt per inch

PERFORMANCE OF A POLYURETHANE CORE SEAL TESTED IN A HYDROSTATIC CHAMBER

By Dennis R. Dolinar,[1] Michael J. Sapko,[2] and Samuel P. Harteis[3]

ABSTRACT

The National Institute for Occupational Safety and Health's Pittsburgh Research Laboratory conducted a full-scale test of a composite polyurethane-aggregate seal in a hydrostatic chamber at the Lake Lynn Experimental Mine. This composite seal consisted of a polyurethane and limestone aggregate core that was formed between two concrete block walls. In the hydrostatic chamber test, water is used to pressurize the seal.

During the test, the maximum average water pressure the seal was able to withstand was 18.9 psi. Further, the seal began to yield at an average water pressure of only 17 psi. At the time of the test, the minimum seal design requirement was 20 psi under 30 CFR[4] 75.335 (2005). Therefore, based on this test, the seal did not meet the regulatory minimum design requirement.

Uniaxial compressive tests conducted on samples from the polyurethane-aggregate core revealed that both the compressive strength and the elastic modulus of the material were much less than that for polyurethane only with a density of 10.0–12.0 lb/ft^3. The significant reduction in the strength and stiffness of the polyurethane-aggregate mixture results from the formation of a soft polyurethane foam around each piece of aggregate. The formation of the soft foam seems to be caused by residual moisture from the aggregate. The moisture also caused the density of the polyurethane in the polyurethane-aggregate mixture to be less than the design requirements. The lower density of the polyurethane in the mixture, along with the formation of zones of pure polyurethane only, resulted in the overall seal density being less than the design requirements. During seal construction, steps were taken to control the moisture, but were not successful.

An analysis of the seal failure showed that the calculated shear stresses at failure and the estimated shear strength of the polyurethane-aggregate mixture are fairly close. This suggests that the strength properties of the polyurethane-aggregate mixture along with a weak zone of poorly bonded aggregate controlled the maximum pressure the seal could withstand.

At the time of the seal testing, the minimum design requirement was 20 psi, as specified at 30 CFR 75.335 (2005). New emergency temporary standards for seal designs were promulgated on May 22, 2007, with a minimum requirement of 50 psi under specified conditions. However, it will be shown that the evaluation of the polyurethane seal performance as designed to meet the older 20-psi criterion can be relevant to the design requirements under the new standards.

---

[1]Lead research mining engineer.
[2]Principal research physical scientist (retired).
[3]Research mining engineer.
Pittsburgh Research Laboratory, National Institute for Occupational Safety and Health, Pittsburgh, PA.
[4]*Code of Federal Regulations.* See CFR in references.

INTRODUCTION

U.S. mine ventilation plans require seals to protect against explosions. They are also used extensively in mining to isolate abandoned areas, fire zones, or areas susceptible to spontaneous combustion. To effectively isolate areas within a mine, a seal should control the methane and air exchange between the sealed and open areas so as to prevent toxic and/or flammable gases from entering the active workings and oxygen from entering the sealed area. A seal must also be capable of preventing an explosion from propagating into or out of the sealed area. Over the years, more than 20,000 seals have been erected in U.S. underground coal mines.

The composite polyurethane-aggregate seal is considered to be an alternative seal design. At the time of the test, alternative seal designs were required to withstand a static 20-psi minimum pressure [30 CFR 75 (2005)]. New emergency temporary standards for seal designs were promulgated on May 22, 2007. Under these standards, the seal strength requirement is 50-psi overpressure when the atmosphere in the sealed area is monitored and kept inert and 120-psi overpressure when the atmosphere is not monitored and not kept inert [72 Fed. Reg.[5] 28795 (2007)]. However, it will be shown that the evaluation of the polyurethane-aggregate seal performance as designed to meet the older 20-psi criterion can be relevant to the design requirements under the new standards. Based on the test results presented in this report, the physical properties of the seal are much less than what is expected from the density of polyurethane used to build the seals. It also proved very difficult to maintain quality control of the strength and elastic properties of the seal material even under the controlled conditions at the Lake Lynn Experimental Mine (LLEM). Further, the results of this investigation are also relevant to the seals designed and installed under the 20-psi criterion and to other seals using the same materials and construction techniques.

Under the old standard, before any new seal design type could be deemed suitable by the Mine Safety and Health Administration (MSHA) for use in underground coal mines, the seal design was generally required to undergo full-scale performance testing at the LLEM [Triebsch and Sapko 1990]. Full-scale explosion testing is very elaborate, time-consuming, costly, and often conflicts with other high-priority research conducted in the LLEM. Further, the explosion method only determined if the seal met the 20-psi criterion; it did not determine the ultimate strength of the seal. With the knowledge of the ultimate strength of the seal, a safety factor for the seal design can be established. Therefore, the National Institute for Occupational Safety and Health (NIOSH) constructed two test chambers within the LLEM where a hydrostatic pressure could be applied to the seals using water. The dimensions of the chambers were 30 ft wide by 15 ft high, and 20 ft wide by 8 ft high. To evaluate the appropriateness of using the hydrostatic chamber to develop the static pressure, a series of tests of various alternate seal designs was subsequently conducted. Data from these chamber studies were used to compare the strength characteristics with the same seal designs previously tested against full-scale 20-psi explosions within the LLEM.

As part of this evaluation program, a composite seal consisting of a polyurethane and limestone aggregate core formed between two concrete block walls was constructed and then tested in the smaller hydrostatic chamber. The design of the seal was based on the 20-psi static pressure requirement. For this seal, the main design requirements are (1) a minimum density of the cured polyurethane of 10 lb/ft^3 and an overall core density of 35 lb/ft^3, and (2) a minimum

---

[5]*Federal Register.* See Fed. Reg. in references.

core thickness of 16 in for seals under 8 ft high with 1 in of thickness added for each foot of height over 8 ft. There is no strength requirement for this seal.

Further, physical property testing of samples from the seal was also conducted. Because a limestone aggregate is used in combination with the polyurethane in the seal construction, the seal consists of sections with a polyurethane-aggregate mixture and sections with only polyurethane. A sampling program was designed to obtain properties of both types of material, as well as to evaluate differences in properties as a result of material anisotropy based on the direction of foam rise.[6] Physical properties included the density and uniaxial compressive strength of the polyurethane and polyurethane-aggregate mixture. This report details the test results of the composite polyurethane-aggregate seal and provides an analysis of those results in terms of the seal's structural behavior.

SEAL CONSTRUCTION AND TESTING

Seal Construction

The constructed seal was 20.4 ft wide by 9.0 ft high with a total thickness, including the forms, of 30 in. Because the entry was higher than 8 ft, the thickness of the polyurethane seal portion was designed by the manufacturer to be 18 in, i.e., 2 in thicker than the standard seal. However, because of some slight bulging of the forms, the actual core seal thickness was 19–20 inches in the middle portion of the seal.

The standard construction practices were followed, and the recommended materials were used for installing this type of polyurethane-aggregate seal. The composite seal tested consisted of two dry-stacked concrete block walls spaced 18 in apart with a polyurethane and limestone aggregate core (Figures 1–2). The concrete blocks used to construct the walls were nominally 16 in by 8 in by 6 in. The back wall was constructed first. After the last block in each row was placed, a wedge was driven between the block and rib to tighten the blocks in place. Wedges were also used between the top row of blocks and the roof. A manhole was left open in the upper right[7] corner of the back wall to allow the back side to be plastered with an MSHA-approved sealant. Once plastering was complete, concrete blocks with MSHA-approved sealant applied to the back side were placed in the manhole until the opening was filled. To complete the back wall at the manhole, boards were used between the top of the blocks and the roof. An MSHA-approved sealant was then used to fill the gap at the roof and ribs. The front wall was constructed similar to the back wall for the first six courses of block. From this point, the blocks were pyramided to the roof so that two blocks were in contact with the roof and wedged in place. An MSHA-approved sealant was then applied to the front side of the outside wall.

---

[6]Upon mixing, rigid polyurethane foam will expand as a result of a blowing agent. The direction of expansion is termed the "rise direction." In this application, the rise direction is generally vertical, except at the top of a lift.

[7]The right or left side of the seal is referenced from the viewpoint of standing outby and facing the seal.

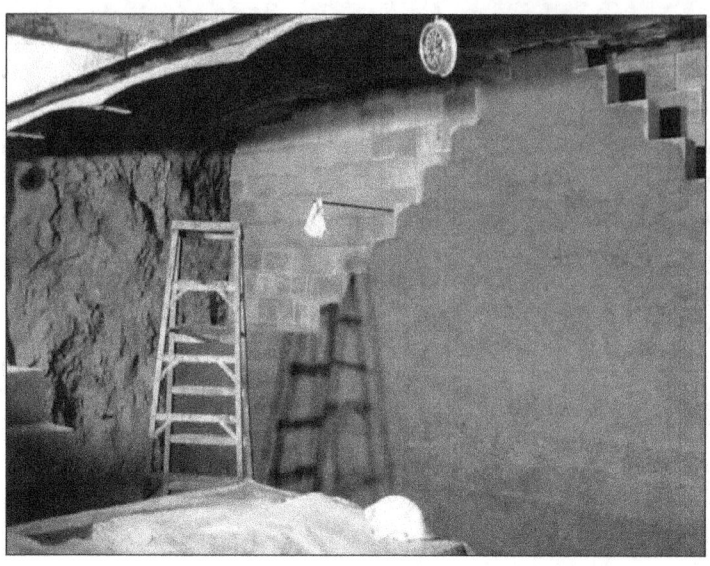

Figure 1.—The dry-stacked concrete block walls comprising the forms for the composite polyurethane seal.

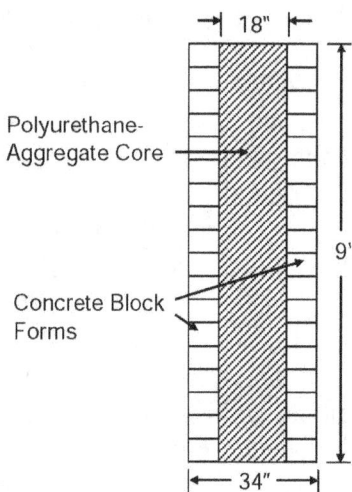

Figure 2.—Vertical cross-section across thickness of the polyurethane-aggregate seal.

Before constructing the inner core, high-density polyurethane was sprayed on the ribs, floor, and around the perimeter of the block walls inside the core area. This was, in part, to provide better adhesion of the seal to the surrounding rock mass and block walls (Figure 3). The improved adhesion, however, only occurs when the polyurethane is still tacky and is limited to the first three lifts. The high-density polyurethane also provided a barrier to protect the low-density foam from moisture or water. For this application, higher-strength polyurethane foam with a density of 70 lb/ft^3 was used. This material was also sprayed along the upper edge of the back wall to improve the seal along the roof line. The high-density polyurethane also fixed the bottom layer of blocks to the floor and was used to saturate the first layer of aggregate to create a good bond with the floor.

4

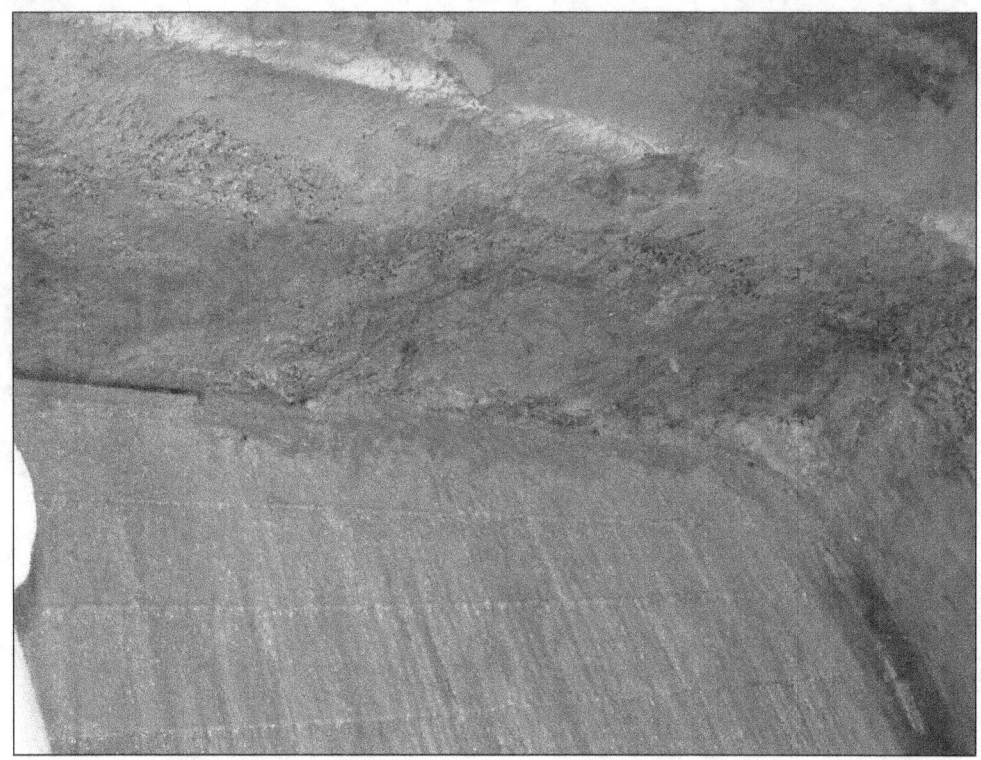

Figure 3.—High-density (70 lb/ft^3) polyurethane sprayed on roof, ribs, and back form wall.

Once the two walls were prepared, the seal core was constructed by placing a limestone aggregate in between the forms and then pumping polyurethane over the aggregate. This process was conducted in a series of lifts. The limestone aggregate is used to add mass to the seal and to reduce the cost. The limestone was sized and graded as AASHTO size number 57 (aggregate size gradation ranges from 0.19 to 1.0 in), which was dried and delivered in plastic lined bags to minimize the possible effects of moisture. The two-component foam was poured into the seal and formulated to have an in-place density of at least 10 lb/ft^3. With the addition of the aggregate, the average seal core density was designed to be a minimum of 35 lb/ft^3. Heating blankets were used to keep the polyurethane at the proper temperature for installation.

The process of developing a lift began by placing a 4-in layer of aggregate at the bottom of each lift, then a polyurethane mixture was poured on top of the aggregate (Figure 4). After the aggregate was placed in a layer, the layer was saturated with polyurethane. The foam would then rise or expand as a result of the blowing agent in the vertical direction. As the polyurethane expanded, the aggregate was carried with and dispersed within the foam. However, depending on the degree of saturation, the polyurethane would expand beyond the aggregate, and a zone of only polyurethane would form a cap at the top of the lift. Once the polyurethane set, a typical lift would be 12–14 in high and consist of an 8- to 12-in thickness of the polyurethane-aggregate mixture and a cap of polyurethane with a thickness of 1–4 in. The cap would generally be 1–2 in thick in the middle of the lift and 2–4 in at the edges. Steps were taken to minimize the thickness of the pure polyurethane cap. Figure 5 shows a typical lift. Eight lifts were used in the seal construction.

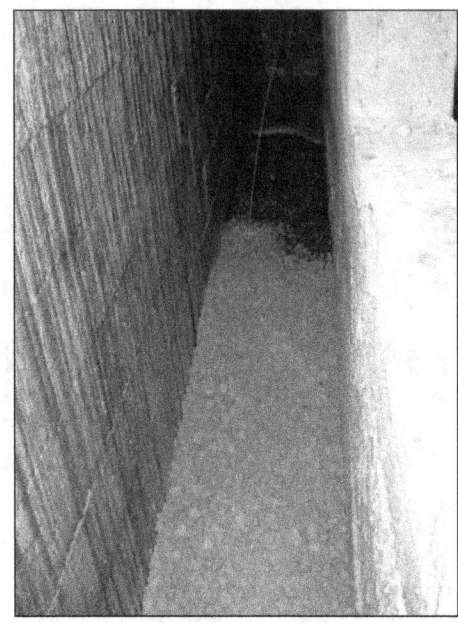

Figure 4.—Polyurethane foam applied on the aggregate at the start of a lift.

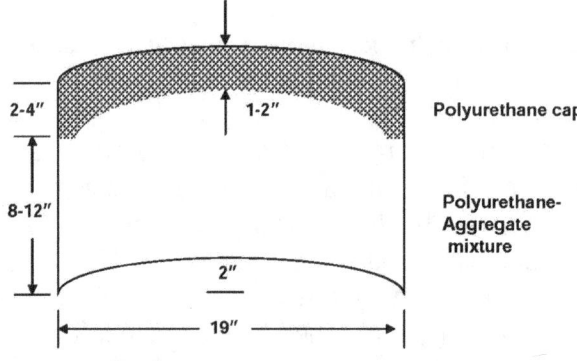

Figure 5.—Cross-section of a typical lift used to form the seal.

Test Setup

Hydrostatic Chamber

Figure 6 shows a diagram of the hydrostatic chamber. The chamber used in this test averages 20 ft wide by 8.0–9.5 ft high by 10 ft deep [Sapko et al. 1999a,b; Sapko and Weiss 2001; Sapko et al. 2003]. The seal was constructed at the front portion of the chamber. A steel frame structure built inside the chamber allows for simulated hitching of the seals. However, for this test the polyurethane seal was not in contact with the steel frame and therefore was not considered hitched. The typical design and installation of these polyurethane-aggregate seals does not require hitching into the surrounding rock.

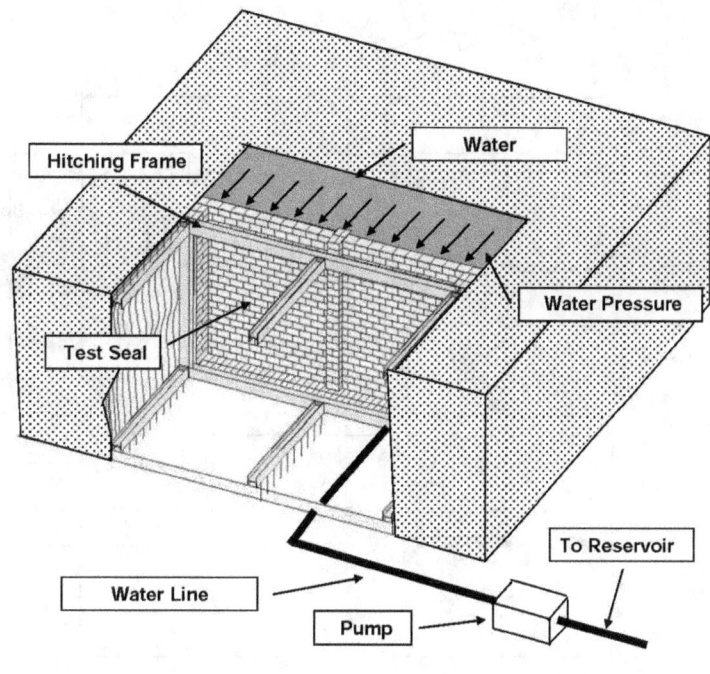

Figure 6.—Schematic of the hydrostatic chamber.

The chamber was connected via remote-controlled air valves to two diesel-driven air compressors that provide 1,000 ft³/min of air. The air compressors are used to conduct the pre- and postexplosion leakage measurements. The chamber is also connected to a 102-hp diesel water pump capable of 1,000 gpm at 90 psi at the chamber inlet with water fed from an underground 130,000-gal reservoir. The pump provided the static horizontal pressure to the seal.

Instrumentation

Eleven linear variable displacement transducers (LVDTs) were used to monitor the displacement of the seal. Figure 7 shows the locations the LVDTs. These spring-loaded LVDTs capable of measuring up to 6 in of displacement were installed on the outside of the seal by attaching them to 2 by 6's that were set between the roof and floor (Figure 8). The LVDTs measured this displacement by generating an output signal of approximately 1.68 V/in. A strain gauge pressure transducer (1,000 Hz) with an internal pressure range of 0–100 psi measured the water pressure behind the seal. This transducer was connected to a pipe placed through the seal and located 6.44 ft above the floor (Figures 7–8). Data from the pressure transducer and LVDTs were recorded at 2,000 samples per second per channel with a WinDaq PC-based data acquisition system.

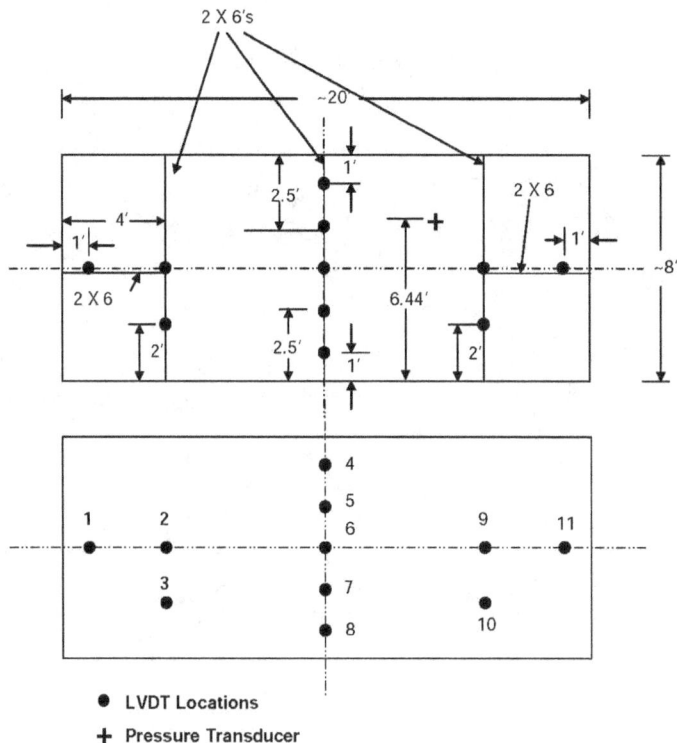

Figure 7.—Locations of the LVDTs and pressure transducer used to monitor displacement of the seal and pressure behind the seal during the test. Nominal dimensions are given for the seal and LVDT locations.

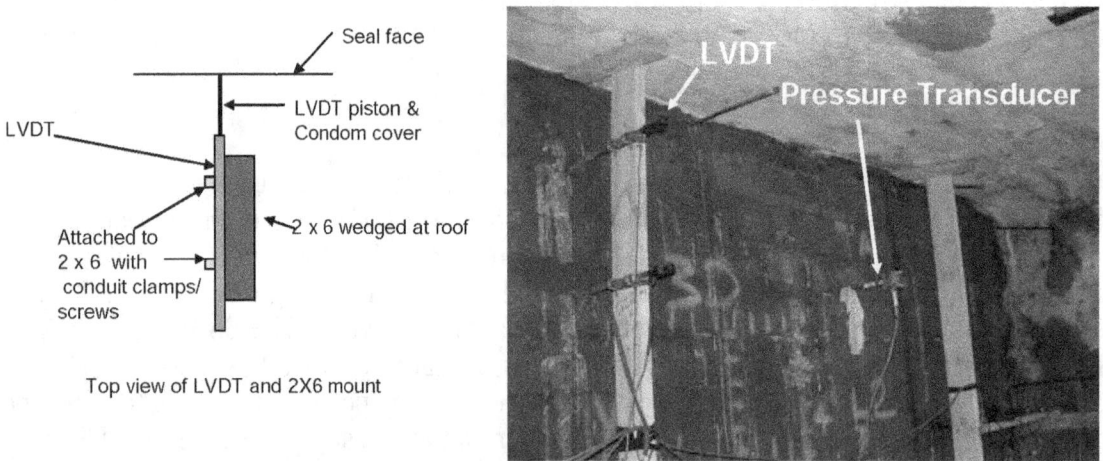

Figure 8.—Pressure transducer and LVDTs used to monitor pressure and deflection during seal test. Schematic of LVDT is shown on the left.

Test Protocol

Before hydrostatically loading the seal, an air leakage test is conducted to confirm that the seal structure met the MSHA-established guidelines. For pressure differentials up to 0.036 psi, air leakage through the seal should not exceed 100 ft^3/min; for pressure differentials over 0.11 psi, air leakage should not exceed 250 ft^3/min. The air leakage test is conducted by pressuring the hydrostatic chamber with compressed air to the guideline pressures. The rate of pressure decay with time is then monitored. The air leakage is calculated from the volume of the chamber and the rate of pressure decay [Sapko et al. 2003]. The results from the air leakage test on this seal prior to the hydrostatic test were within the guidelines.

Following the leakage test, the seal would be hydrostatically loaded to 20 psi at the pressure transducer (6.44 ft above the floor). When this pressure was achieved, pumping would be stopped and the water drained from behind the seal. The seal would then be subjected to a second air leakage test to determine if the seal could still function for ventilation purposes. If the seal passed the second air leakage test, the seal would be hydrostatically loaded to a pressure where the seal failed structurally.

Hydrostatically loading the seal creates a differential pressure between the top and bottom of the seal. For a 20-psi pressure at the transducer, the pressure is 18.9 psi at the top of the seal and 22.9 psi at the bottom. The average pressure across the seal is 20.9 psi.

Test and Test Results

Figure 9 shows the flow rates and water pressures generated during the test. In the initial phase, the pumping rate was 250–350 gpm. Once the chamber behind the seal was filled, the remaining portion of the test then took 13–14 min to complete.

Figure 10 shows the pressure and the displacements with respect to time for the five LVDTs placed along the vertical center line of the seal. The responses of the LVDTs along the horizontal center line are shown in Figure 11, and the responses of the two LVDTs just off the horizontal center line are shown in Figure 12. During the initial pressurization to about 11 psi, the pressure-time curve showed a stairstep behavior. This behavior resulted from adjustments to the rate of pressurization using a pressure relief value at the pump. At just over 16 psi at about 3,100 sec into the test, significant leakage began to occur through the seal. This resulted in several sudden pressure drops just before reaching the maximum pressure. A maximum pressure of 18 psi at about 3,250 sec into the test was achieved at the transducer. Just past the peak pressure, a large amount of displacement occurred at all LVDT locations over a short period of time (Figures 10–12). After the maximum pressure was reached and the pressure dropped to about 11 psi because of leakage, the flow rate was increased to 800 gpm to determine if a higher pressure could be achieved. Although the pressure did increase to 14 psi with the higher pumping rate, there was an accompanying rapid increase in the seal deflection. This resulted in severe leakage from the seal and a rapid pressure drop to about 8 psi. The maximum seal deflection of at least 6 in at the center of the seal was recorded at this time. However, several of the LVDTs had reached their maximum stroke limit of 6 in. The pumping was then halted and the water was allowed to drain from behind the seal at 3,650 sec into the test. As the pressure dropped, there was some rebound of the seal with up to 2 in of displacement recovered near the center. However, there was still nearly 4 in of displacement that was not recovered by the end of monitoring.

9

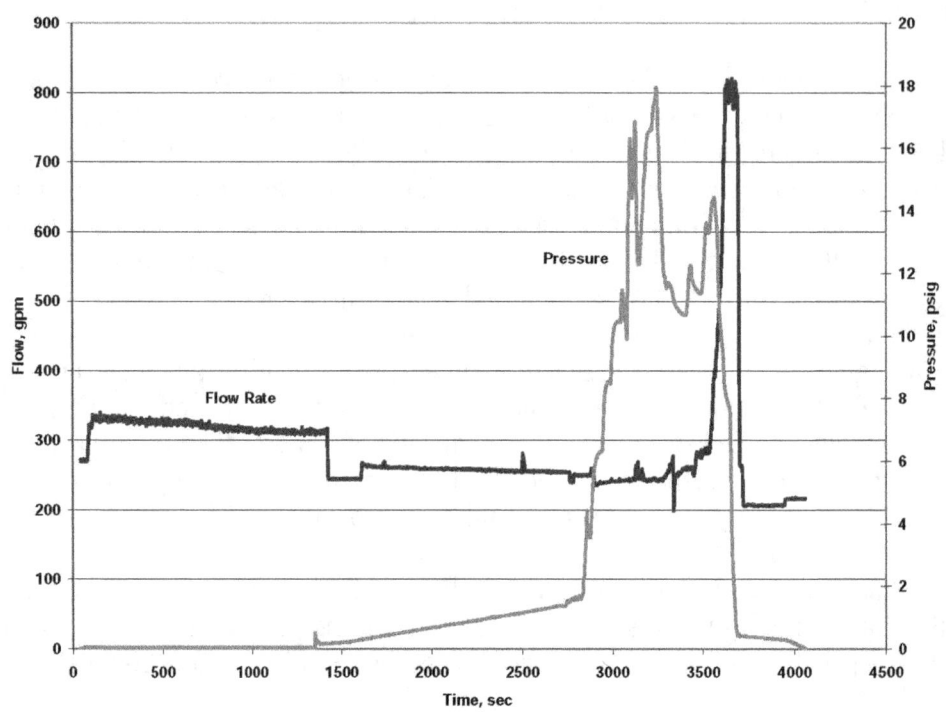

Figure 9.—Water pressure and flow rate versus time during seal test.

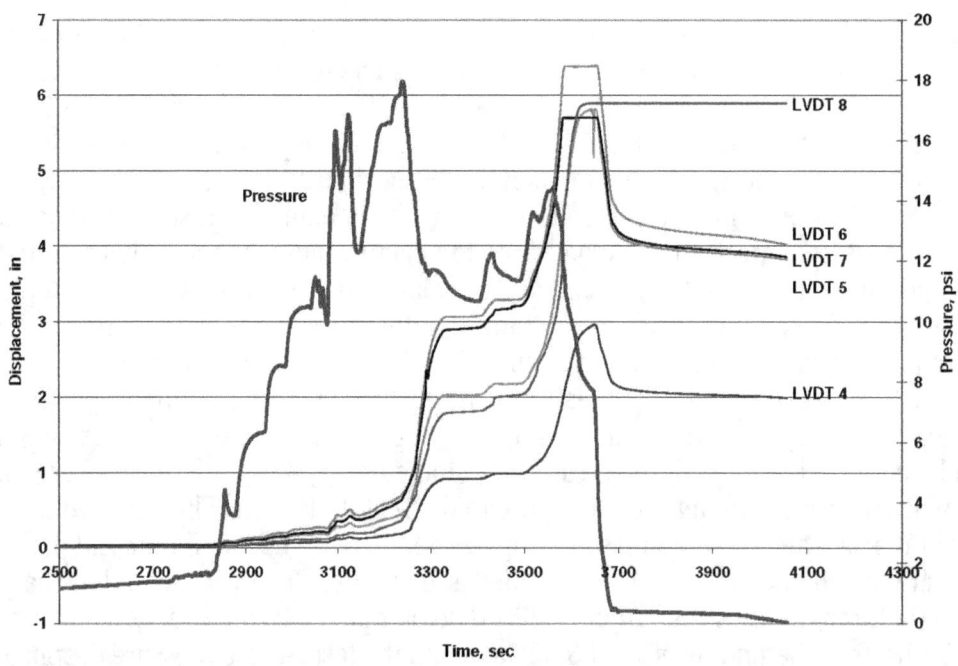

Figure 10.—Displacement for LVDTs along the vertical center line of the seal and pressure recorded versus time.

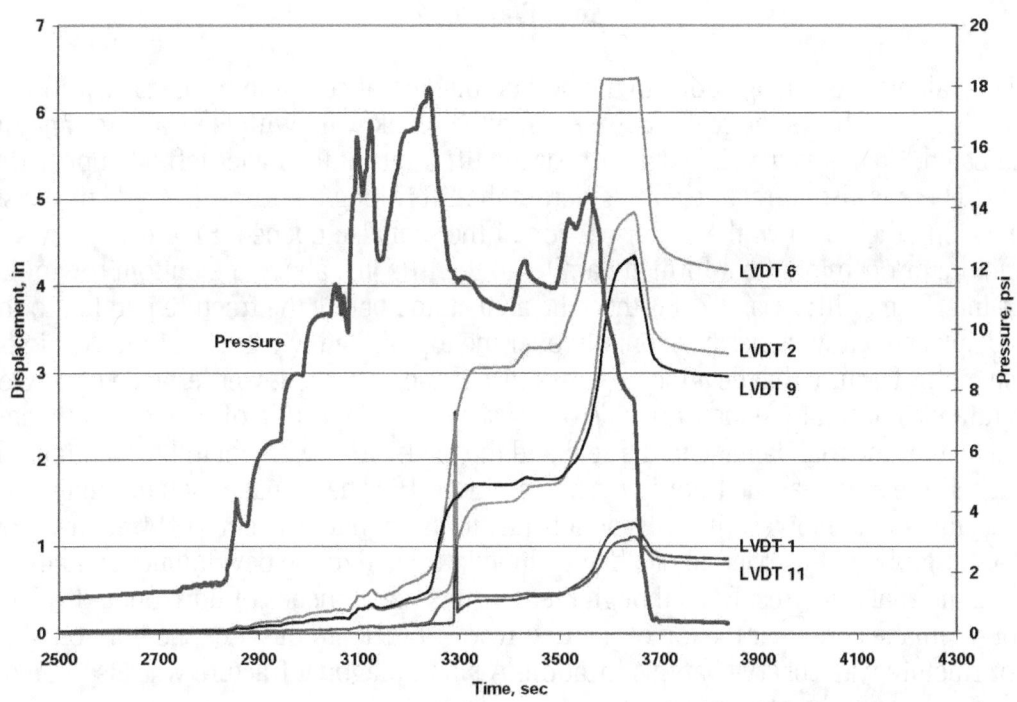

Figure 11.—Displacement for LVDTs along the horizontal center line of the seal and pressure recorded versus time.

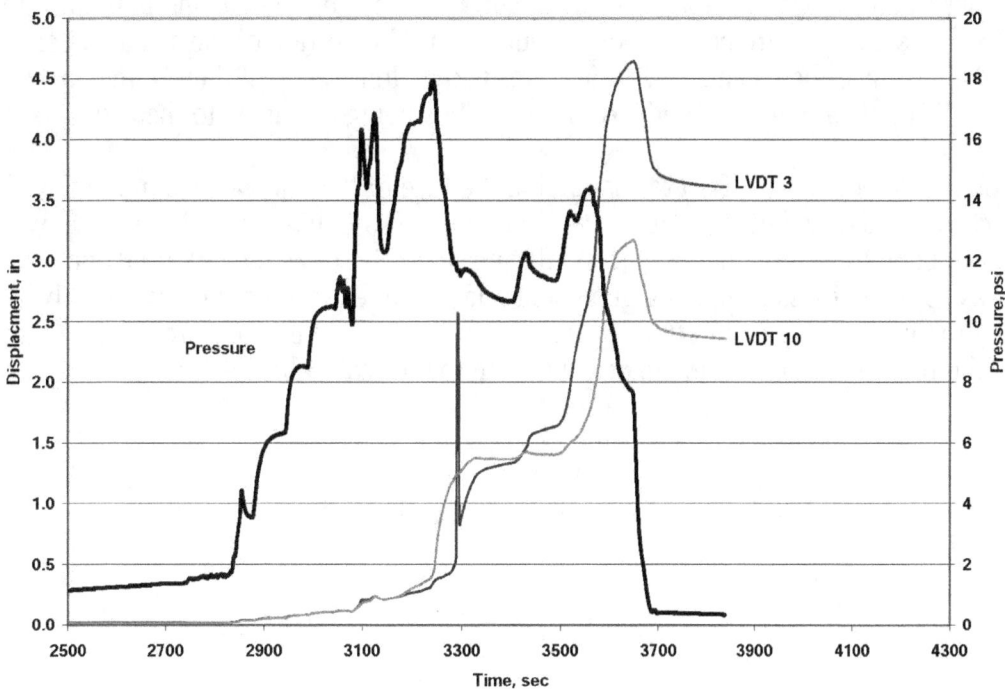

Figure 12.—Displacement for LVDTs just off the horizontal center line near the ends of the seal and pressure recorded versus time.

11

Seal Damage

To evaluate the damage done to the polyurethane seal core, the front stack wall was removed. Figure 13 shows the seal after removing the block wall, with the fractures and open joints indicated. Fractures developed at or near the lift joints at the lower left and upper right side of the seal. There is also a fracture cutting across the lifts along the lower left side of the seal. The joints along the lifts near the center portion of the seal also opened. Figure 14 shows the major fracture or open joint that formed parallel to the lifts just above the bottom row of blocks along the interface of lifts 1 and 2. Further, the area at and below the fracture parallel to the lift line was displaced a few inches horizontally over the top of the lowest row of block. Figure 15 shows the major fracture that developed across lifts 1 and 2 on the lower left side of the seal. This fracture was open along the front side of the seal core. A portion of the polyurethane was excavated so that internal damage to the seal and the back block wall could be examined. Internal damage to the seal near the floor is shown in Figure 16. The damage includes major near-vertical fractures in the lowest lift. This area is just to the right of the external fracture shown in Figure 15. Essentially, the external damage is directly related to the development and movement along these internal fractures. Even though there were several inches of horizontal displacement of the polyurethane core over the top of the first row of blocks in this area, no horizontal shear surface or fracture was observed at this location. A small diagonal fracture was also noted in the upper left quadrant of the seal (Figure 13).

Another zone of damage and deformation occurred near the roof and extends across most of the right side of the seal (Figure 13). In exposed portions of this damaged zone, there is high concentration of aggregate with very little polyurethane to lift the aggregate and to act as a binder (Figure 17). The seal below the fractured zone was displaced outward.

Other fractures opened along the joined surfaces between the top and bottom of the lifts (Figure 13). This occurred in the lifts from the upper middle portion of the seal and below and involved the interfaces between lifts 1 to 5. Cores taken along some of these joint surfaces reveal that the joint is open only to the middle of the seal, thus being restricted to the tension side of the seal (Figure 18).

Also, two long narrow fissures parallel to the face of the seal were found in the poly-urethane caps. These fissures were about 24–30 in long, 2–3 in high, and about 0.5 in wide. They seem to have been caused by thermal effects during foam rise or as the polyurethane was setting. Possibly, as a result of less heat being generated due to the reduced volume of the polyurethane in the polyurethane-aggregate mixture, no fissures were noted in the mixture. These voids, however, did not seem to be related to or contribute to the seal failure.

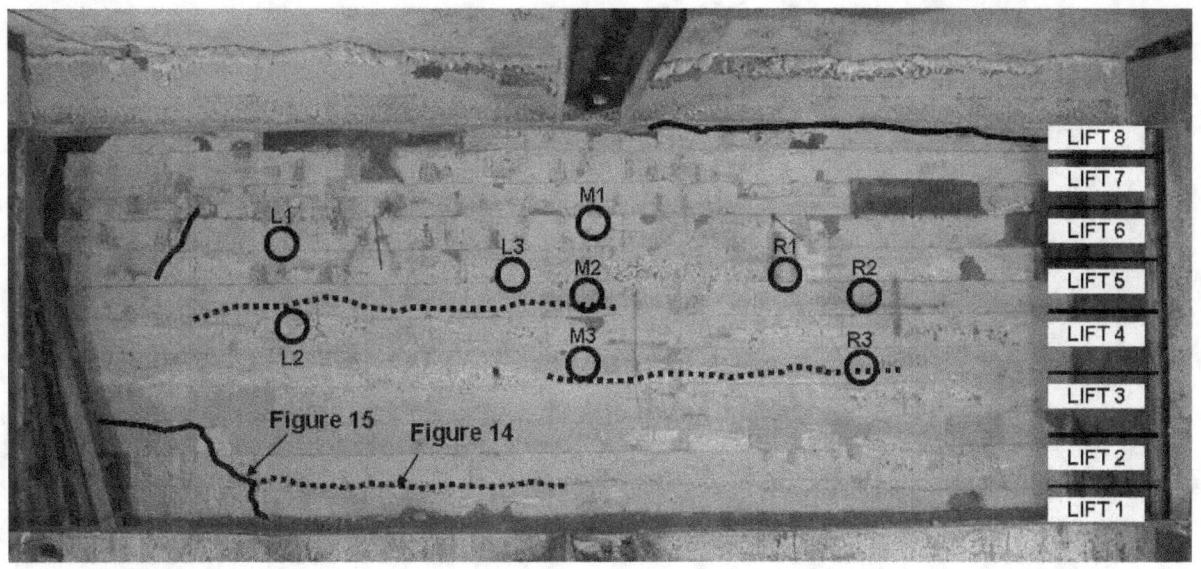

Figure 13.—Damage observed in polyurethane core after removing block form. Fractures in seal are indicated with solid lines; open joints along lifts are indicated with dashed lines. Circles denote where core was obtained for compressive tests.

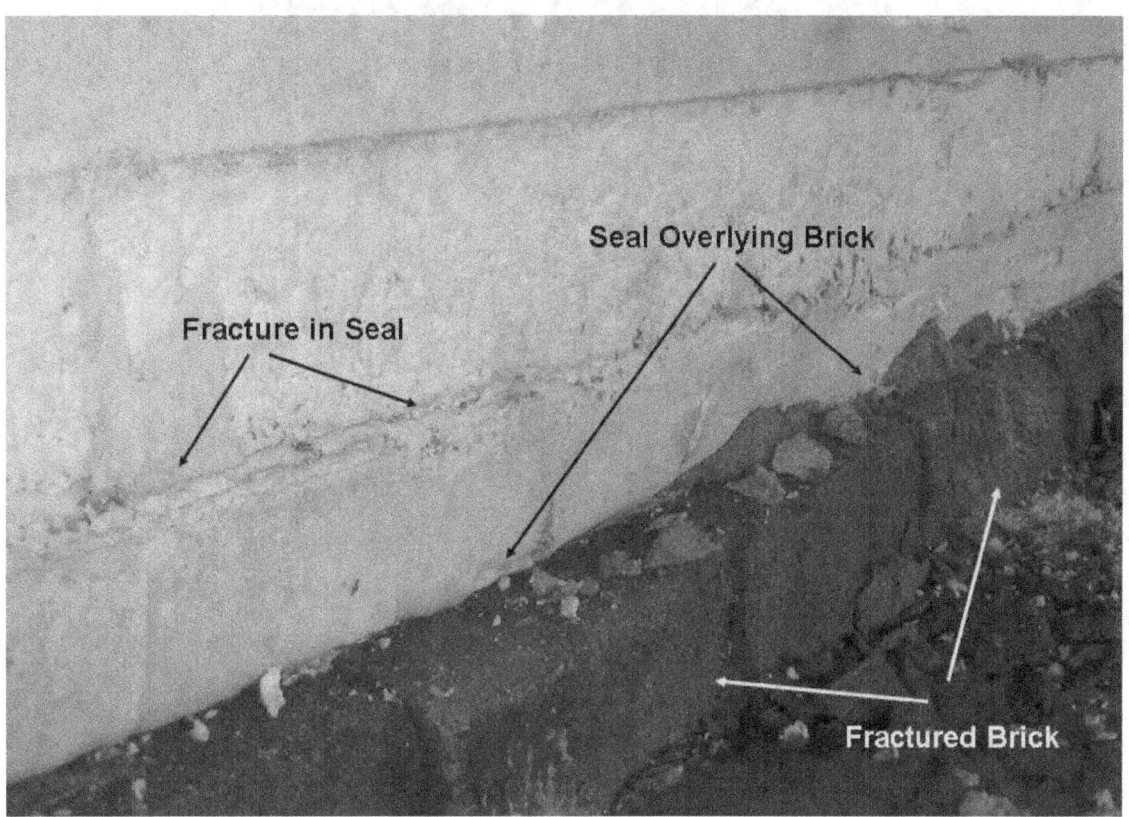

Figure 14.—Closer view of damage observed along lower left side of polyurethane seal along top of bottom row of blocks. Seal has displaced about 2 in over the top of the blocks. The fracture or open joint is along the interface of lifts 1 and 2.

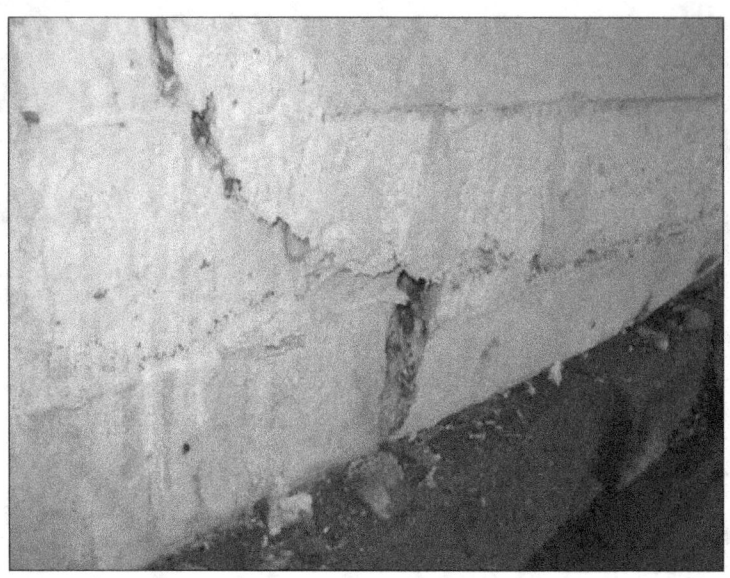

Figure 15.—Fracture and damage observed along lower left side of polyurethane seal along top of bottom row of blocks.

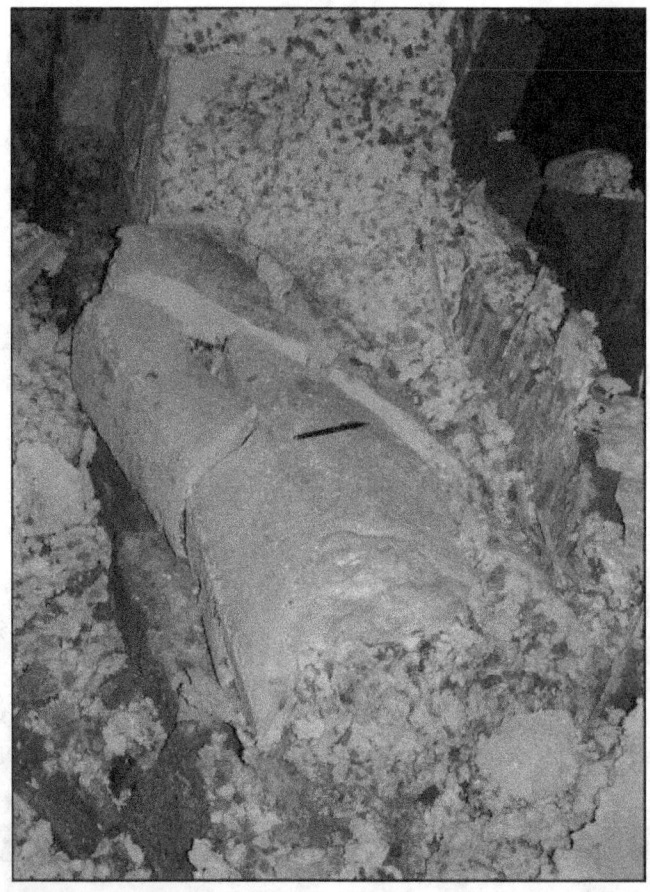

Figure 16.—Internal damage along lower left side of polyurethane seal just above of the bottom row of blocks.

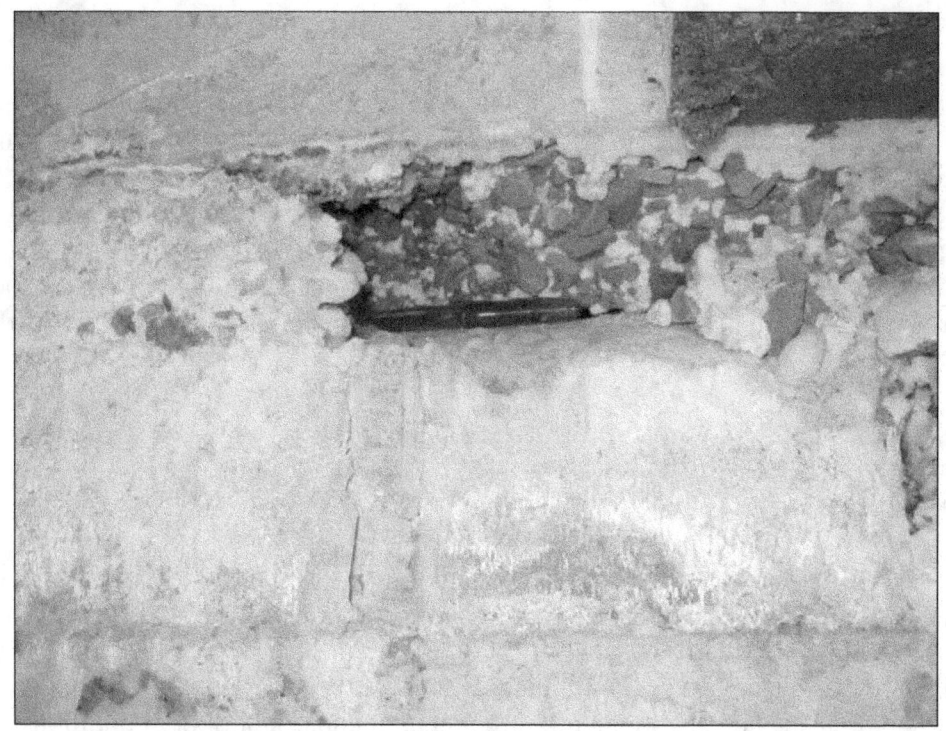

Figure 17.—High concentration of aggregate that is poorly bonded with polyurethane observed along upper right side of seal.

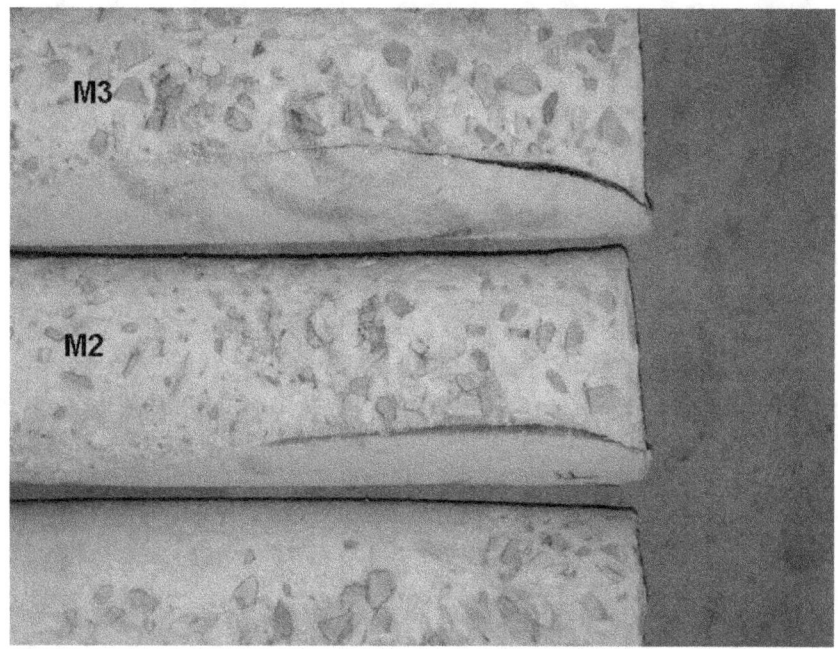

Figure 18.—Separation along the interface between lifts observed in 6-in-diam core drilled horizontally. The right side of the cores is the front side of the seal.

SEAL MATERIAL PROPERTIES

To evaluate the material properties of the seal, uniaxial compressive tests were conducted on cylindrical samples taken from the seal. From these tests, compressive strengths could be determined and an elastic modulus calculated. The sample densities were also measured. These properties were evaluated to determine if the materials in the seal, installed under field conditions at the LLEM, met the seal construction requirements. Further, the results of the tests could be used to analyze the seal performance. However, the targeted design requirements for this type of seal were based in large part on the density of the seal and not on the strength or stiffness properties.

Sampling and Testing

Lift Composition

Because of the addition of the aggregate in the seal, there are two zones that develop in a lift: a zone consisting of a mixture of polyurethane and aggregate, and a polyurethane cap (Figure 5). By volume, about 80% of the lift is composed of the polyurethane and aggregate mixture where the polyurethane cap is 1–4 in thick. However, the reported results from previous tests on the polyurethane and aggregate mixture prepared under laboratory conditions indicated there was no apparent reduction in the elastic modulus when the aggregate was added [Sawyer 1999]. In the present testing program, samples from a seal constructed under field conditions would be tested. Therefore, the testing program was designed to evaluate the materials to determine physical properties developed under field conditions.

Test Procedures and Measurements

Cylindrical specimens were tested in uniaxial compression to determine the strength of the seal materials. These specimens were obtained by either drilling the seal in situ or by drilling of larger sections of the seal that had been brought back to the NIOSH Pittsburgh Research Laboratory after the seal was dismantled. For the polyurethane and aggregate mixture, because the nominal aggregate size was 1 in, 6-in- diam samples were used. For the polyurethane cap, both 2- and 6-in-diam specimens were prepared.

The ends of the cylindrical specimens were cut parallel and perpendicular to the axis with a diamond saw to a length that resulted in a length-to-diameter ratio of one for the specimens [ASTM 2004b].[8] No other surface preparation was done to the ends of the specimens. A length ratio of one was used to accommodate the aggregate size of the polyurethane-aggregate mixture.

The uniaxial compressive tests were conducted on a servocontrolled load frame with the tests being conducted in displacement control. During the tests, both the load and displacement were recorded. To measure the displacement, the main activator LVDT for the load frame was used. The specimens were strained 30%–50% over a 10–15 min period. This timeframe is similar to that of the seal test.

---

[8]According to ASTM standards for testing rigid cellular plastics, the length-to-diameter ratio of the samples should not exceed one. The only specifications for the ends of the samples are that they are parallel and perpendicular to the sides.

From the uniaxial compressive tests, the compressive strength, elastic modulus, and proportional limit were determined. The compressive strength is the stress at the yield point or, where there is no distinct yield point, the stress at 10% strain [ASTM 2004b]. The elastic modulus is determined from the near linear portion of the stress-strain curve below the proportional limit.

The density of the specimens was determined by two methods. For regularly shaped specimens, the weight and dimensions were measured directly according to ASTM standards [ASTM 2004a]. For irregularly shaped specimens, a water displacement test was used [ASTM 2004c].

Sampling

Specimens for the compressive tests were obtained by two methods: in situ drilling of the seal and laboratory drilling of large sections removed from the seal. In situ 6-in-diam cores were obtained by drilling horizontally into the seal. Figure 13 shows the location of the coreholes with respect to the lifts. Because the polyurethane cap and polyurethane-aggregate mixture interface was intersected in a significant number of the cores, only cores from four of the holes (L2 (lift 4), L3 (lift 5), M1 (lift 6), R1 (lift 5)) were prepared and tested (Figure 18). However, the length of the cores allowed for two 6-in-long samples to be tested from these four holes. The resulting samples were tested in the direction perpendicular to foam rise and provided properties of the polyurethane-aggregate mixture.

Several large sections of the seal were brought back and cored in the laboratory. The sections were either one or two full lifts in height. Six-inch-diameter cores orientated both perpendicular and parallel to foam rise were drilled. For the polyurethane and aggregate mixture, samples were obtained from lifts 2 and 5. For the polyurethane cap, 6-in-diam samples were also obtained from lifts 4 and 5. However, these samples had a length of only about 2 in because of the cap thickness. Further, 2-in-diam cores from the polyurethane cap orientated both perpendicular and parallel to foam rise were drilled from lift 4.

Seal Material Properties

Table 1 shows the results of the uniaxial compressive tests on the cores of the polyurethane-aggregate mixture. Test results include samples from lifts 2, 4, 5, and 6. Figure 19 shows typical stress-strain curves for the mixture for samples tested both perpendicular and parallel to foam rise. Table 2 shows the strength and deformation properties for the polyurethane cap with samples from lifts 4 and 5. Typical stress-strain curves for samples from the polyurethane cap tested perpendicular and parallel to foam rise are shown in Figure 20. A summary of the results is given in Table 3.

For the polyurethane and aggregate mixture, the average density is 33.7 lb/ft^3. Parallel to foam rise, the average compressive strength is 41 psi with an elastic modulus of 1,187 psi. Perpendicular to foam rise, the average compressive strength is 32 psi with an elastic modulus of 635 psi.

For the polyurethane cap, the average density is 11.0 lb/ft^3. The average compressive strength is 210 psi parallel to foam rise and 240 psi perpendicular to foam rise. The average elastic modulus is 5,810 psi parallel to foam rise and 7,753 psi perpendicular to foam rise.

Table 1.—Results of uniaxial compressive tests on polyurethane-aggregate mixture samples

Sample	Lift	Density, lb/ft³	Diameter, in	Length, in	Compressive strength, psi	Strain,[1] %	Proportional limit, psi	Elastic modulus, psi
PARALLEL TO FOAM RISE								
L2VC	2	28.2	5.675	6.13	26	10	13	550
L2VA	2	27.5	5.675	6.13	35	10	18	1,012
L2VB	2	32.5	5.675	6.13	39	10	22	1,215
Average	—	**29.4**	**5.675**	**6.13**	**33**	**10**	**18**	**926**
PERPENDICULAR TO FOAM RISE								
L2HA	2	28.5	5.675	6.13	24	10	9	452
L2HB	2	28.1	5.675	5.92	23	10	9	410
Average	—	**28.3**	**5.675**	**6.03**	**24**	**10**	**9**	**431**
PERPENDICULAR TO FOAM RISE								
L2 A	4	42.8	5.875	6.125	31	10	7	715
L2 B	4	35.2	5.875	6	41	10	16	906
Average	—	**39.0**	**5.875**	**6.06**	**36**	**10**	**12**	**811**
PARALLEL TO FOAM RISE								
L5VA	5	32.2	5.675	6.25	42	10	20	1,042
L5VB	5	31.7	5.675	6.13	51	10	29	1,954
L5VC	5	50.3	5.675	6.13	42	10	21	1,181
L5VD	5	34.7	5.675	6.38	55	10	24	1,355
Average	—	**37.2**	**5.675**	**6.22**	**48**	**10**	**24**	**1,383**
PERPENDICULAR TO FOAM RISE								
L5HA1	5	31.2	5.675	6.19	32	10	12	743
L5HA2	5	34.4	5.675	5.92	37	10	16	861
L5HB1	5	28.2	5.675	6.06	36	10	12	559
L5HB2	5	30.3	5.675	6.06	28	10	15	583
L3 A	5	37.9	5.875	6.063	40	10	17	789
L3 B	5	40.1	5.875	6	36	10	12	655
Average	—	**33.7**	**5.742**	**6.05**	**35**	**10**	**14**	**698**
PERPENDICULAR TO FOAM RISE								
M1 A	6	37.7	5.875	6.063	20	10	8	246
R1 A	6	33.4	5.5	6.125	26	10	12	432
R1 B	6	30.5	5.5	6	38	10	15	900
Average	—	**33.8**	**5.625**	**6.063**	**28**	**10**	**12**	**526**

[1]Strain at the compressive strength.

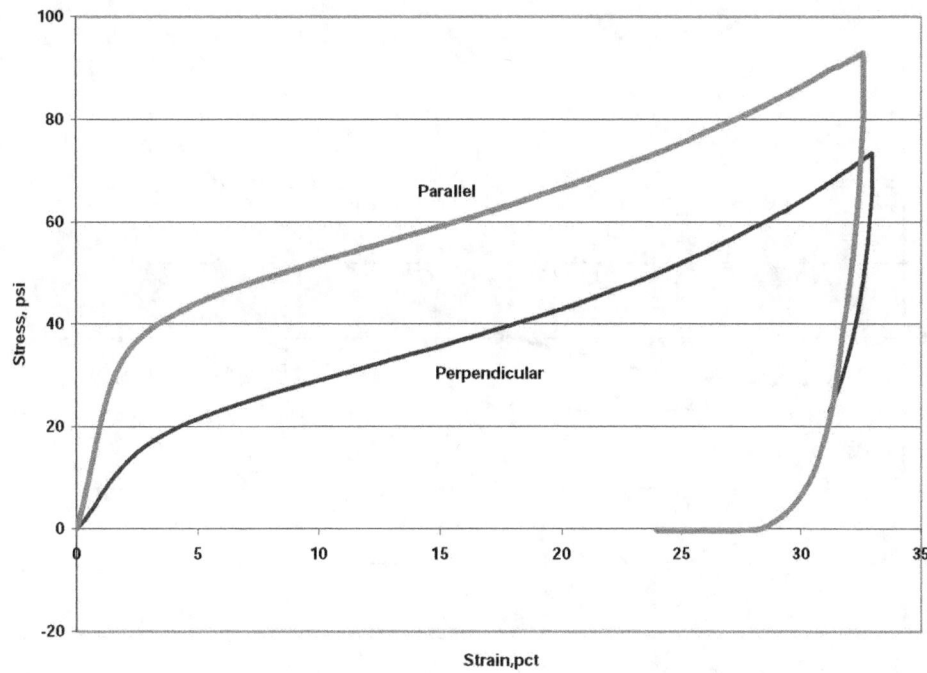

Figure 19.—Typical stress-strain curves developed from uniaxial compressive tests on polyurethane-aggregate mixture tested both perpendicular and parallel to the direction of foam rise.

Table 2.—Results of uniaxial compressive tests on the polyurethane lift caps from the polyurethane seal

Sample	Lift	Density, lb/ft³	Length, in	Diameter, in	Compressive strength, psi	Strain,[1] %	Proportional limit, psi	Elastic modulus, psi
PARALLEL TO FOAM RISE							
L4VC1	4	11.4	1.98	1.995	215	7	140	7,372
L4VC2	4	11.2	1.99	1.995	210	6	160	7,495
L4VC3	4	11.2	1.98	1.995	220	6	170	7,577
L4VC4	4	11.2	1.96	1.995	210	10	150	5,081
L4VC5	4	11.2	2.03	1.995	200	6	155	6,607
Average	—	**11.2**	**1.99**	**1.995**	**211**	**7**	**155**	**6,826**
L4VCA	4	10.6	2.393	5.675	205	10	160	5,509
L4VCB	4	10.77	1.793	5.675	215	10	175	4,792
L4VCC	4	11.02	2.005	5.675	200	10	160	5,018
L4VCD	4	11.06	1.522	5.675	210	10	170	4,614
L5VCA	5	11.04	2.069	5.675	210	10	160	4,731
L5VCD	5	11.08	1.955	5.675	215	10	155	5,112
Average	—	**10.93**	**1.956**	**5.675**	**209**	**10**	**163**	**4,963**
PERPENDICULAR TO FOAM RISE							
L4HC1	4	11.2	2.156	1.995	215	10	90	5,390
L4HC2	4	10.8	1.99	1.995	260	5	220	8,584
L4HC3	4	11.3	2.2	1.995	250	10	210	8,020
L4HC4	4	10.5	2.07	1.995	215	5	180	7,746
L4HC5	4	10.9	1.99	1.995	260	5	215	9,026
Average	—	**10.9**	**2.08**	**1.995**	**240**	**7**	**183**	**7,753**

[1]Strain at the compressive strength.

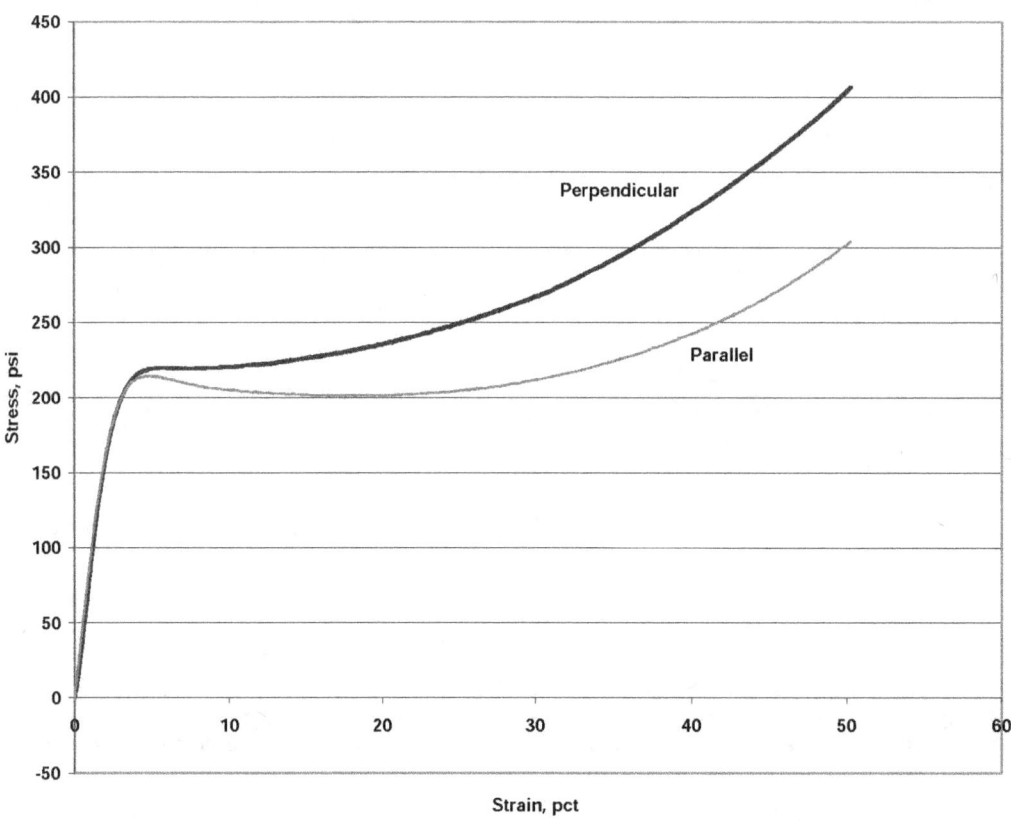

Figure 20.—Typical stress-strain curves developed from uniaxial compressive tests on polyurethane-only cap of lift.

Table 3.—Summary of results of uniaxial compressive tests on samples from the polyurethane seal

Direction of foam rise	No. of samples	Density, lb/ft³	SD, lb/ft³	Compres-sive strength, psi	SD, psi	Strain,[1] %	Propor-tional limit, psi	SD, psi	Elastic modulus, psi	SD, psi
POLYURETHANE-AGGREGATE MIXTURE										
Perpendicular	13	33.7	4.8	31.7	6.9	10	12.3	3.3	635	208
Parallel	7	33.8	7.7	41.4	7.7	10	21	5	1,187	423
Average	**20**	**33.7**	**5.8**	**35.1**	**9.1**	**10**	**15.4**	**5.7**	**828**	**396**
POLYURETHANE LIFT CAP										
Parallel	11	11.07	0.22	210	6.3	8.6	160	10	5,810	1,200
Perpendicular	5	10.94	0.32	240	23.2	7	183	54	7,753	1,411
Average	**16**	**11.03**	**0.25**	**219.4**	**19.4**	**8.1**	**167**	**32**	**6,417**	**1,535**

SD   Standard deviation.
[1]Strain at the compressive strength.

Change in Foam Characteristics and Properties in the Polyurethane and Aggregate Mixture

The physical characteristics of some of the polyurethane foam were different from the rigid foam in the polyurethane cap, as were the properties of the remaining foam in the mixture. The differences in physical characteristics occurred in the foam surrounding each piece of aggregate where a soft foam layer formed. This formation is clearly associated with the aggregate and may be caused by residual moisture from the aggregate. Residual moisture can affect the polyurethane in two ways [Zhang 2006]. It can cause the formation of additional carbon dioxide gas beyond the specified formulation and result in lower-density polyurethane near the moisture source. Further, the stoichiometric balance between the two components (the isocyanate and polyalcohol used to form the polyurethane) will be upset with the extra moisture. This could cause some of the polyalcohol component not to react, and thus the foam could become softer in the vicinity of the residual moisture.

The soft foam can easily be deformed with finger pressure. The thickness of the soft layers measured about 0.06–0.15 in. Essentially, the material has different characteristics from the rigid foam and now behaves as soft foam. Moving away from the aggregate, the foam becomes rigid, similar to the polyurethane cap. Therefore, the polyurethane-aggregate mixture consists of aggregate surrounded by soft foam that is dispersed in a matrix of rigid foam.

The density and the variation of the density of the polyurethane in the mixture caused by the residual moisture can be used as a measure of the changes in the polyurethane foam and to determine if the design requirements were achieved. The estimated amount of soft foam in the mixture can also be determined from the density. For rigid polyurethane, there is a strong, direct correlation between density and the strength and stiffness [DuPont 1987; Piping Technology & Products 2008]. However, it is assumed that the soft foam has little or no strength regardless of the density, and the amount of soft foam would then have a significant effect in reducing the overall strength and stiffness of the mixture.

To determine the density, the aggregate was removed from a 6-in-diam cylindrical sample from the polyurethane-aggregate mixture from lift 2. The combined sample had a volume of 88.2 in^3 with a weight of 1.77 lb, resulting in a density of the mixture of 34.7 lb/ft^3. The weight of the aggregate was 1.56 lb with a density for the aggregate of 160 lb/ft^3. The density of the aggregate was measured by using a water displacement method [ASTM 2004c]. Based on weight and density, the volume of the aggregate in the sample was calculated to be 16.9 in^3. The weight of the polyurethane foam was 0.21 lb with a volume of 71.3 in^3. The calculated foam density in the mixture is 5.1 lb/ft^3. This is much less than the design requirement of 10.0 lb/ft^3. Based on this sample, the percent by volume of the aggregate in the mixture is 19.2, and the percent by volume of the polyurethane foam is 80.8.

The amount of softer foam that has formed in the mixture can be estimated from the potential difference in the density between the two foams. Table 4 shows the densities of various samples of the soft, rigid, and combined foams. These foam densities were determined using a water displacement method [ASTM 2004c]. The samples were obtained by taking pieces of the foam from a lift and removing the aggregate. Some of the foam samples were further dissected to separate the soft and rigid foam. Because of this process, measurements were made on small, highly irregular samples.

**Table 4.—Densities of soft, rigid, and combined foam samples
taken from the polyurethane-aggregate mixture[1]**

Sample	Weight, g	Specific gravity	Density, lb/ft^3	Location
RIGID FOAM				
L4-R	1.05	0.15	9.31	Middle lift 4
L3-R	1.52	0.14	8.81	Lift 3
L3/L4-R	3.01	0.15	9.26	Lift 3/Lift 4
L3/L4-R	3.71	0.16	9.83	Lift 3/Lift 4
Average	—	**0.15**	**9.30**	—
SOFT FOAM				
L3-Sa	2.18	0.06	4.02	Middle lift 3
L5-S	1.71	0.08	4.89	Lift 5
L4-S	1.66	0.09	5.38	Lift 4
L3-Sb	2.33	0.07	4.55	Lift 3
Average	—	**0.08**	**4.71**	—
COMBINED RIGID AND SOFT FOAM				
L3-Ca	4.98	0.09	5.54	Lift 3
L3-Cb	5.31	0.12	7.18	Middle lift 3
L4-Ca	2.37	0.11	7.01	Bottom lift 4
L4-Cb	6.6	0.14	8.54	Lift 4
L5-C	5.78	0.10	6.31	Lift 5
Average	—	**0.11**	**6.92**	—

[1]Densities were measured by water displacement method.

The density of the soft foam was measured at 4.7 lb/ft^3 and the density of the rigid foam at 9.3 lb/ft^3. The combined density was 6.9 lb/ft^3. Based on these densities, the polyurethane portion of the polyurethane-aggregate mixture is composed of about 50% soft foam. It must be recognized that these densities are based on small grab samples. Further, the amount of soft foam is dependent on the amount, size, and gradation of the aggregate. These parameters vary through a lift. Also, the density of the combined foam samples as measured by this technique is higher than the apparent density of 5.1 lb/ft^3 based on a much larger sample. The higher density results from the penetration of water into the foam during the water displacement tests caused by voids along the surface. With the small, highly irregular samples used, the surface area is quite large compared to the volume; therefore, the density determined by water displacement can be higher than the apparent density. However, the assumption is made that the porosity along the sample surfaces is approximately the same for the two types of foam, and the densities measured by this method can be used to estimate the percent of each type of foam. Regardless of these assumptions and sampling issues, it is clear that the amount of soft foam in the mixture is substantial.

The formation of soft foam in a polyurethane seal has also been noted from a seal that was destroyed in a mine explosion [MSHA 1996]. In the 1996 explosion at the Oasis Mine in West Virginia, three polyurethane seals were destroyed and one partially destroyed. The seals contained a 16-in-wide core composed of polyurethane and aggregate. From the explosion, the seals were blown apart into primarily small pieces. Based on the examination of a small piece of the seal that was primarily polyurethane, MSHA [1996] reported that "[t]his polymer could be compressed or broken by hand." However, as a result of the hazardous conditions at the site and in the mine, there were no further site visits to examine the failed seals.

ANALYSIS OF SEAL PERFORMANCE

Analysis of Seal Material Properties

Based on the results of the seal material testing, the properties of the two sections of a lift are significantly different. The two sections include the polyurethane cap and the polyurethane-aggregate mixture, with the mixture comprising about 80% of a lift and of the polyurethane seal (Figure 5).

The cap consists of polyurethane with a density of about 11.0 lb/ft^3. This does fall above the designed minimum density of 10.0 lb/ft^3 for the polyurethane. In general, the stress-strain curves show the type of performance expected from rigid polyurethane foam with this density (Figure 20) [DuPont 1987; Huber and Gibson 1988; Piping Technology & Products 2008]. Initially, there is an elastic portion to the curve that is nearly linear. This is followed by a sharp flattening of the curve or even a slight drop in the stress as the foam structure collapses. Beyond the compressive strength, the stress-strain curve continues to rise, although at a much reduced rate with a nearly plastic material behavior. Further, there does not seem to be a large difference in the compressive strength between the vertical and horizontal direction. Typically, the collapse or compressive strength may be 30%–50% lower in the direction perpendicular to foam rise [Huber and Gibson 1988]. This anisotropic behavior results from a polyurethane cell structure that is more elongated in the direction of foam rise. In this case, the compressive strength is about 14% higher in the direction considered to be perpendicular to foam rise. The strength properties indicate either that the aspect ratio of the cells is close to one, where there is no cell elongation, or the orientation of the cell structure is not vertical and horizontal [Hawkins et al. 2005]. At the top of a lift, the foam that forms the cap will be free to expand not only in the vertical direction, but also in the horizontal direction, which could result in a variation of the orientation of the cell structure.

The density of the polyurethane-aggregate mixture that was sampled is about 34 lb/ft^3. Based on the estimated volumes and densities of the polyurethane cap and polyurethane-aggregate mixture, the overall density of the core seal is 29 lb/ft^3. The minimum design density for the seal is 35 lb/ft^3. To meet the minimum density requirement, the polyurethane-aggregate mixture would need to have a density of 40 lb/ft^3. In part, the lower measured density of the mixture could be due to sampling. However, the lower density of the polyurethane foam in the mixture could account for a significant portion of this difference.

The polyurethane-aggregate mixture has significantly lower compressive strengths and deformation properties than the cap with only polyurethane. The compressive strengths and elastic modulus are only about 15% of those of the polyurethane cap. This significant reduction in properties is the result of the formation of the soft foam around the aggregate. Further, there is not a sharp transition from the pre- to the postcompressive strength regions on the stress-strain curves (Figure 19).

The reduction in strength results from the rigid foam forming a stiff structural matrix around the soft foam and aggregate, where the soft foam may comprise up to 50% by volume of the polyurethane in the mixture. However, the soft foam contributes little to the compressive strength, and the aggregate surrounded by the soft foam could be approximated as a hole or void until the matrix collapses. Essentially, the rigid foam matrix structure must support the load. This rigid matrix does provide some initial stiffness to the specimen until the rigid foam in the matrix structure collapses. Because the aggregate and soft foam are distributed through the samples and the lift, the strength is based to a large extent on the matrix structure and not the percent by volume of the soft and rigid foam.

Based on the measured compressive strengths and elastic moduli from the two orthogonal directions, the polyurethane-aggregate mixture seems to be anisotropic. In the direction of foam rise, the compressive strength is about 31% higher and the elastic modulus about 87% higher than perpendicular to foam rise. It is possible that the rigid foam within the polyurethane-aggregate mixture may be anisotropic, thus resulting in a higher strength and stiffness in the direction of foam rise. However, this effect is small compared to the reduction in properties from the addition of the aggregate.

The density of the polyurethane foam in the mixture is a further indication of the changes that occurred with the addition of the aggregate. The foam density in the mixed zone is 5.1 lb/ft^3. It is much lower than the cap density of 11.0 lb/ft^3. This in part reflects the formation of a large amount of the soft foam. However, as measured by the water displacement method, the density of the rigid foam within the mixed zone may have a lower density (9.3 lb/ft^3) than the poly-urethane in the cap. Because of the porosity, this measured density (9.3 lb/ft^3) may be over-estimated in making a comparison with the density measured for the cap. Essentially, the rigid foam within the mixed zone could have a correspondingly lower compressive strength than the foam cap based on the density.

Clearly, the formation of the soft foam is closely associated with the aggregate, as is the overall lower density of the foam in the mixture. It is assumed these changes are occurring because of residual moisture on the aggregate. The aggregate was added to provide additional mass; however, there was also a significant reduction in the compressive strength and stiffness of the polyurethane-aggregate mixture due to the addition of the aggregate. The importance of this compressive strength is that once it is exceeded, the material will exhibit nearly plastic behavior.

Seal Failure

Figure 21 shows the pressure-displacement curve for LVDT 6 located at the center of the seal. The pressure used is that at the pressure transducer. From 0 to 4 psi, the curve is linear, indicating a linear elastic behavior for the seal. From 4 to 16 psi, the curve shows some nonlinear characteristics, possibly associated with inelastic behavior that is time-dependent. Fitting a line from 4 to 16 psi, the decrease in slope indicates some softening of the seal. However, from 16 to 18 psi a significant change in behavior occurs. This was accompanied by a larger increase in visible leakage from the seal. Again, fitting a line between the pressure peak at 16 psi and the maximum pressure at 18 psi shows a further and significant softening of the seal. This suggests that structural damage to the seal was taking place after the pressure reached 16 psi at the pres-sure transducer. Therefore, 16 psi can be considered the yield strength for the seal. This calcu-lates to an average pressure across the seal of about 17 psi based on the stress distribution of the hydraulic load.

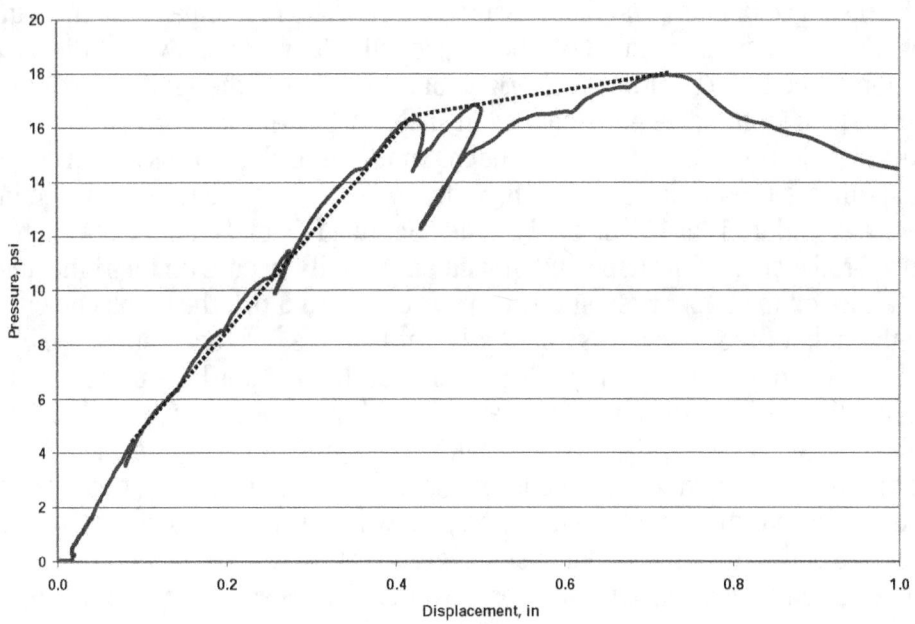

Figure 21.—Pressure-displacement curve for LVDT 6 at the center of seal shows the behavior of the seal. General slopes of curves are indicated by dashed lines.

Based on the average pressure on the seal of 17 psi at yield and the seal surface area of 184 ft^2, the total force on the seal was about 450,000 lb. With a seal thickness of 18 in and assuming no contribution from the forms, the calculated shear stress along the boundary at yield was 35.3 psi. Assuming the seal acts as a plate with simply supported edges, a center deflection at yield of 0.46 in, an elastic modulus of 828 psi for the polyurethane-aggregate mixture, and a seal thickness of 18 in, the maximum stress due to bending is 3.2 psi.[9] The shear stresses are an order of magnitude higher than the bending stresses. Therefore, the yielding is probably the result of the shearing stresses developed near the boundaries.

The maximum pressure that the seal withstood at the pressure transducer was 18 psi. As shown in Figures 10–12, at that point there was a large increase in displacement with a sudden drop in pressure. This occurred as the seal failed and the pumping could not keep up with the leakage. Further loading at an increased pumping rate did not achieve a higher maximum pressure, but did significantly increase the deflection and water leakage. Essentially, the 18-psi static pressure can be considered the pressure where the seal structurally failed. When this occurred, the stress was 16.9 psi at the top of the seal and 20.8 psi at the bottom. This calculates to an average stress across the seal of 18.9 psi. This is below the 20-psi criterion mandated by the Code of Federal Regulations at the time of the test [30 CFR 75 (2005)].

---

[9]For a seal simply supported at the edges, the maximum stresses from bending will be in the middle of the seal, with the back of the seal core in compression and the front in tension. If the seal edges are assumed to be fixed, the maximum stress from bending would increase to 10.5 psi. This stress is still much lower than the shear stress. With the edges fixed, the maximum stresses from bending are in the center of the long side of the seal. The back of the seal would be in compression and the front in tension at the maximum stress location.

From the observed damage and the pressure and displacement measurements, an understanding of how the seal may have failed can be developed. Figure 22 shows the displacement versus the location of the LVDTs along the horizontal center line of the seal for various pressures. The lines on the graph indicate the change in shape of the seal for a given pressure. The heavy line (third from left) is the deflection at the maximum transducer pressure of 18 psi. All curves past this point are for a failed seal. At the initiation of failure, there is a change in the geometry of the seal. Failure is also indicated by the continued displacement even with a pressure drop. However, the change in shape and movement initially occurs on the right side of the seal. After the failure on the upper right side, at a pressure of 13.5 psi, the displacement at the location 6 ft to the right of the center was initially larger than the displacement at the center. Little or no additional movement is seen on the left side of the seal until the pressure has dropped to 10.9 psi. Figure 23 shows the displacement versus time for LVDTs 2 (left side), 6 (center), and 9 (right side). There is about a 40-sec delay before the increase in displacement is seen on the left side as opposed to that on the right side and center. The main damage observed along the right side of the seal is near the top where the aggregate was not well bonded with the polyurethane (Figures 13 and 17). A major leak also developed at this location (Figure 24). This high concentration of poorly bonded aggregate can be considered a construction flaw.

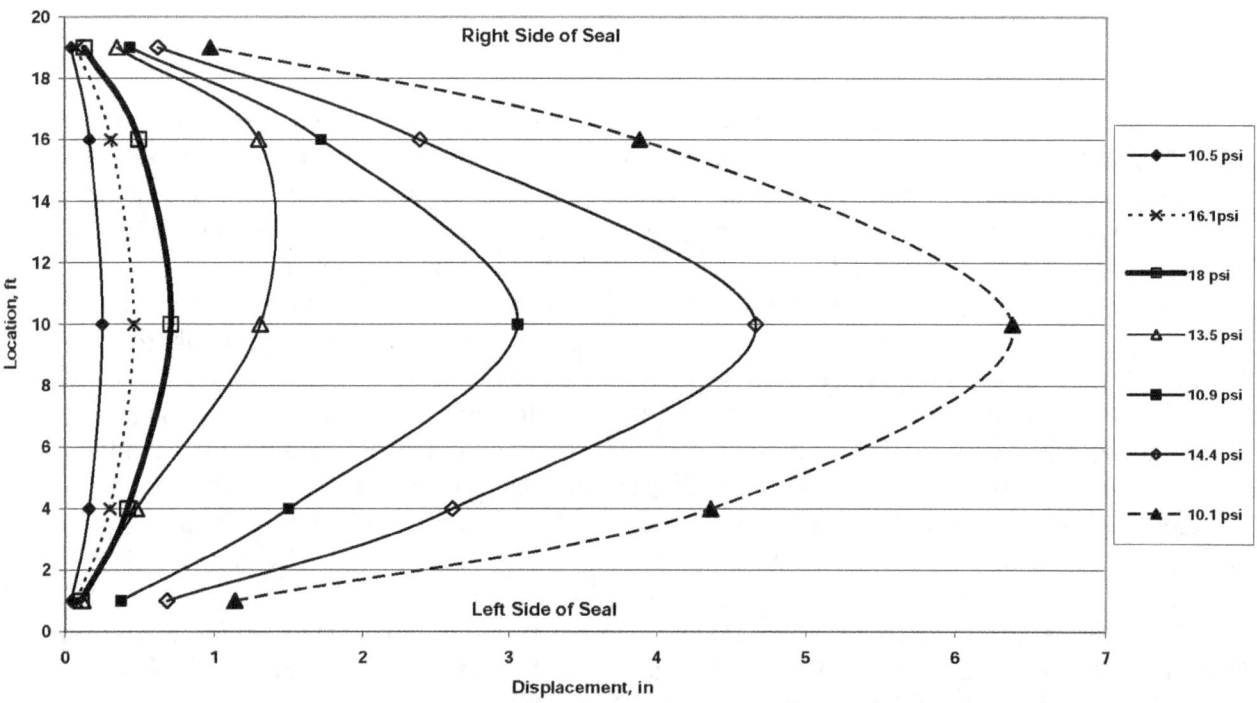

Figure 22.—Displacements along horizontal center line of the seal show the change in shape of the seal during the test for a given transducer pressure. Curves to the right of the 18-psi line represent the behavior after the peak pressure was achieved.

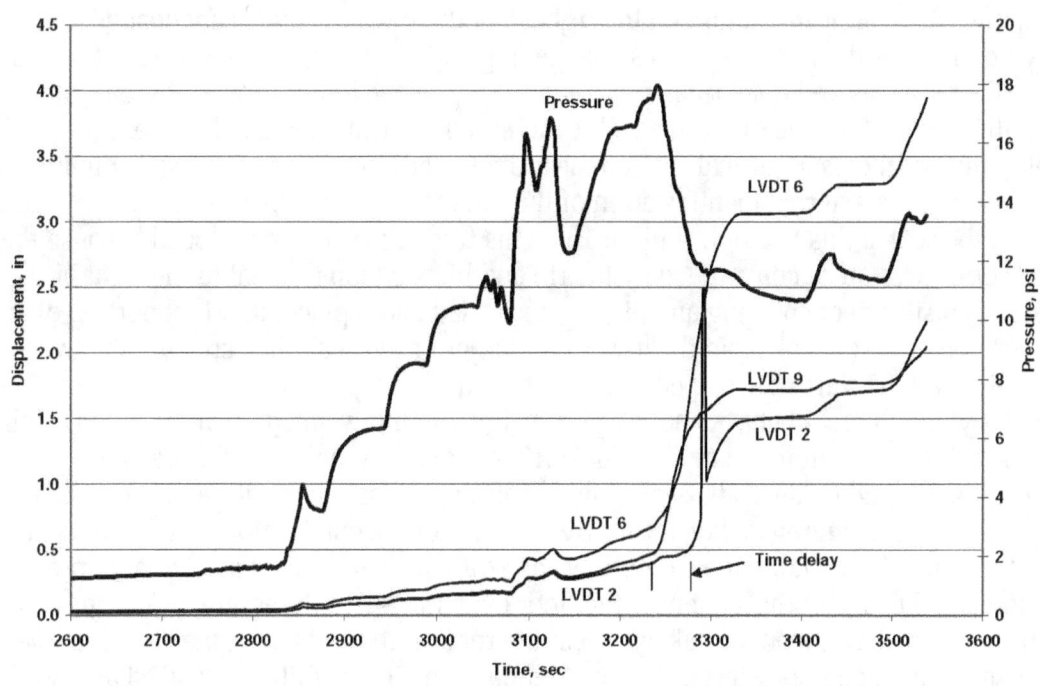

Figure 23.—Displacements measured on the left side (LVDT 2), center (LVDT 6), and right side (LVDT 9) of seal showing the 40-sec delay in the reaction of the left side when the seal failed.

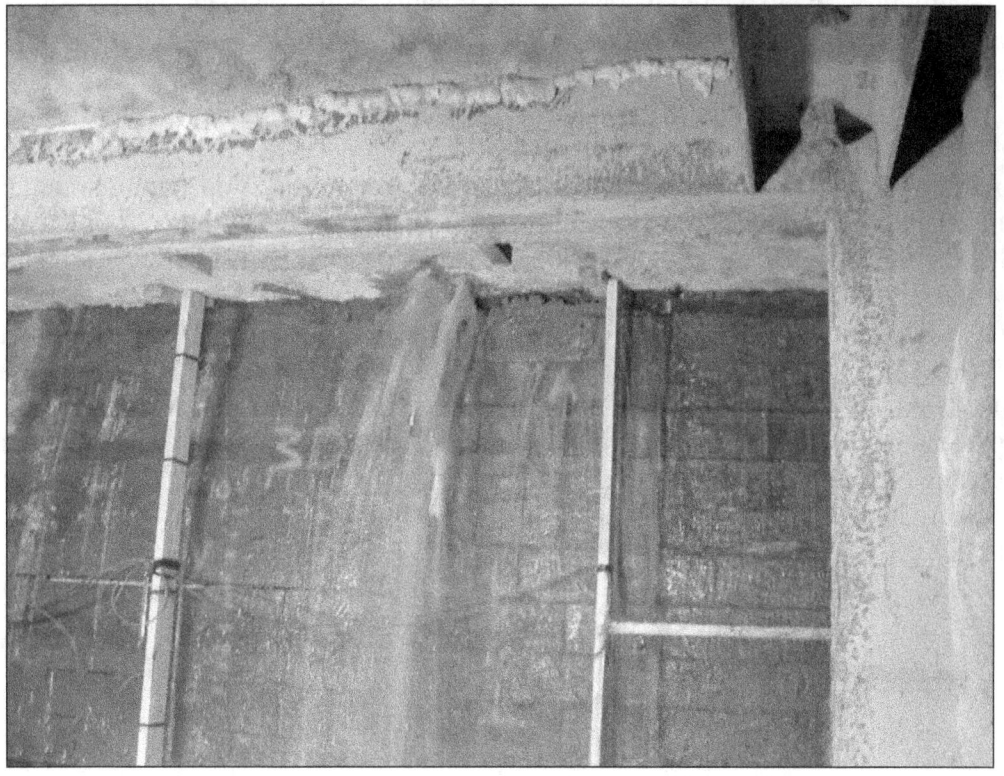

Figure 24.—Water leakage observed from failure zone along upper right side of the seal.

About 40 sec after the failure on the right side, there was a significant change in the geometry on the left side of the seal. This change in geometry probably developed as a result of increased shear stresses and displacements along the top of the bottom row of blocks due to the failure on the upper right side of the seal. This increased shearing and displacement resulted in the development of the near vertical fracture near the lower left corner of the seal (Figures 13 and 15). This was the external manifestation of the internal fractures that extended across the thickness of the seal at this location (Figure 16). This fracture system developed because the lower left corner was more constrained by the rib and blocks than the seal to the right of the fractures. When sufficient shearing and displacement had taken place, the right portion of the seal was torn or sheared away from the lower left corner of the seal, thus creating the fractures. Mostly likely these fractures developed at or just past the peak pressure.

After yield, the seal behaves nearly plastically with a low stiffness, indicating that the seal is approaching maximum strength. With sufficient displacement, the failure was initiated near the roof on the right side of the seal probably as a result of shear failure through the seal along a poorly bonded aggregate layer. Shortly after, failure occurred along the lower center and left side of the seal. Essentially, the strength of the seal material was not sufficient to prevent deformation and damage in this area near the floor even though the pressure was dropping. Although there may have been a weak area near the roof on the right side, the area near the floor did not seem to be much stronger. Further, even though the initial failure occurred at a weakened zone, the seal was in yield, indicating that the seal was close to the maximum strength even without a weak point.

After the seal had failed structurally, the water flow rate was increased to 750 gpm and there was a subsequent increase in pressure to 14.5 psi. However, the seal could not sustain this added pressure, resulting in a large increase in deformation and a sharp drop in pressure to less than 8 psi. At this point, the fracture through the seal on the lower left side would probably have been fully developed (Figure 15).

Following yield and failure, the seal was subjected to a significant increase in displacement and bending. Approximately 95% of the displacement occurred after yield and 90% after failure. As a result of the bending of the seal, the horizontal interfaces opened between lifts toward the center of the seal. These interfaces were only open to the middle of the seal, indicating that the joint opened because of tension caused by bending. The interfaces do not appear to have affected the failure. The open joints, however, indicate that the interfaces between the lifts were weaker than the polyurethane-aggregate mixture in tension. This suggests that the polyurethane is not bonding well to itself after curing. Much of the damage to the seal along the top of the lower row of blocks probably occurred in the postfailure period (Figure 15). The large seal displacements and the opening of the joint along the interface of lifts 1 and 2 at this location were probably caused by shearing along the top of the bottom row of blocks. This shearing created a sharp bend in the seal core just above this location that resulted in the opening up of the interface.

During the test there was only a little over 1 in of deflection recorded by the two LVDTs just 1 ft from each rib. This indicates that there was little or no slippage of the seal along the rib boundaries. To a large extent, the seal was restrained at the ribs.

28

Shear Failure and Strength of the Seal

The assumption is made that the seal was in yield because of the shear stresses developed from the water pressure. Further, the failure seems to have occurred in shear near the upper right corner and lower left boundary. Therefore, an estimate can be made of the shear stresses along the boundary at failure. These average shear stresses can then be compared to the strengths measured for the seal material.

Based on the average pressure on the seal of 18.9 psi at failure and the seal surface area of 184 ft^2, the total force on the seal was about 500,000 lb. With a seal thickness of 18 in and assuming no contribution from the forms, the calculated shear stress along the boundary at failure was 39.4 psi.[10] Because of how the failure initiated, this may represent the shear strength along the upper right side of the seal, a zone of poorly bonded aggregate that can be considered a construction flaw. However, the seal was in yield before the failure occurred at this weakened zone; therefore, the shear strength of the seal without this construction flaw may not be that much higher.

Since the failure occurred through the polyurethane-aggregate mixture, the strength properties of this material are used to evaluate the strength of the seal. From the tests, only a uniaxial compressive strength was measured and not the shear strength. However, a similar reduction in the shear strength that occurred with the compressive strength from that of a pure polyurethane sample is assumed.

Strength equations have been developed that can be used to estimate the expected strength of a rigid polyurethane from the density [DuPont 1987; Piping Technology & Products 2008]. For the compressive strength, the equation is

$$C_o = 12.77D^{1.416} \tag{1}$$

where C_o = compressive strength, psi,
and D = density of polyurethane, lb/ft^3.

For the shear strength, the equation is

$$S_o = 14.9D^{1.077} \tag{2}$$

where S_o = shear strength, psi.

These equations are for the strength in the direction of foam rise or in the strong direction. Further, although these equations were developed for specific polyurethane formulations, they can be used as general equations showing the effect of the density on strength.

The average compressive strength for the polyurethane-aggregate mixture is 35 psi (Table 3). In this analysis, no consideration is being given to the affects of foam anisotropy since there is such a large reduction in strength with the addition of the aggregate. Based on the average compressive strength for the polyurethane-aggregate mixture, the density of polyurethane foam that would result in the same compressive strength can be calculated. From the above

---

[10]The maximum bending stresses for the seal core are for a fixed-end beam 2–3 times less and for a simply supported beam 6–10 times less than this calculated shear stress.

29

equations, a foam density of 2 lb/ft^3 would result in a compressive strength of 34 psi and a shear strength of 31 psi.[11]

The estimated shear strength of 31 psi for the polyurethane and aggregate mixture is certainly within the same magnitude range as the calculated shear stresses developed at failure. Therefore, shear failure through the polyurethane-aggregate mixture could have occurred. Essentially, when the stresses in the seal exceeded the strength of the polyurethane-aggregate mixture, which had changed because of the residual moisture from the aggregate and the construction flaw, the seal failed. Thus, the properties of the polyurethane-aggregate mixture and the construction flaw determined the maximum pressure that the seal could withstand.

Contribution of the Concrete Block Walls
to the Strength and Stiffness of the Seal

One can ask whether the dry-stacked concrete block wall forms increased the strength or stiffness of the seal and thus could be an important element in maintaining the structural integrity of the seal. The possible effects of the forms on the stiffness can be evaluated from the pressure and deflection data prior to failure. Figure 25 shows the deflection of the seal along the vertical center line for different water pressures before and after failure.

In the following analysis, the seal performance with both a fixed and simply supported edge will be evaluated. For the fixed-edge condition, the assumption is made that the middle portion of the seal will act as a beam in bending with the edge constraints provided by the ribs sufficiently removed so their effects can be ignored [Obert and Duvall 1967]. However, for a plate with simply supported edges, the error in using the beam equations is larger and may not be sufficiently accurate. Therefore, both the plate and beam equations will be used for this case. The actual deflections can then be compared to those calculated from a bending beam or plate. Considering only the seal core, the calculations are as follows: beam length is 9 ft, plate length is 20.4 ft and plate width is 9 ft, and thickness for both is 18 in. The elastic modulus was then adjusted so that the calculated deflection in the center of the beam or plate matched the measured deflection. Table 5 shows the calculated deflection at locations where the measurements were made and the resulting elastic modulus. Values were calculated for both fixed-end and simply supported beams and for a plate with simply supported edges. To develop the same amount of deflection at the center of the seal for the range in pressure from 4.6 to 16.1 psi, the elastic modulus for the fixed-end beam ranges from 22,500 to 32,500 psi and for a plate with simply supported edges from 84,000 to 125,000 psi.

---

[11]The 90% confidence interval for the shear strength equation at a density of 2 lb/ft^3 is from 20 to 50 psi. However, these confidence intervals are based on testing different formulations of the polyurethane where the confidence levels are the variation between the formulations. If the strength of the formulation is less than the average strength for a given density, it will be less than the average for all densities.

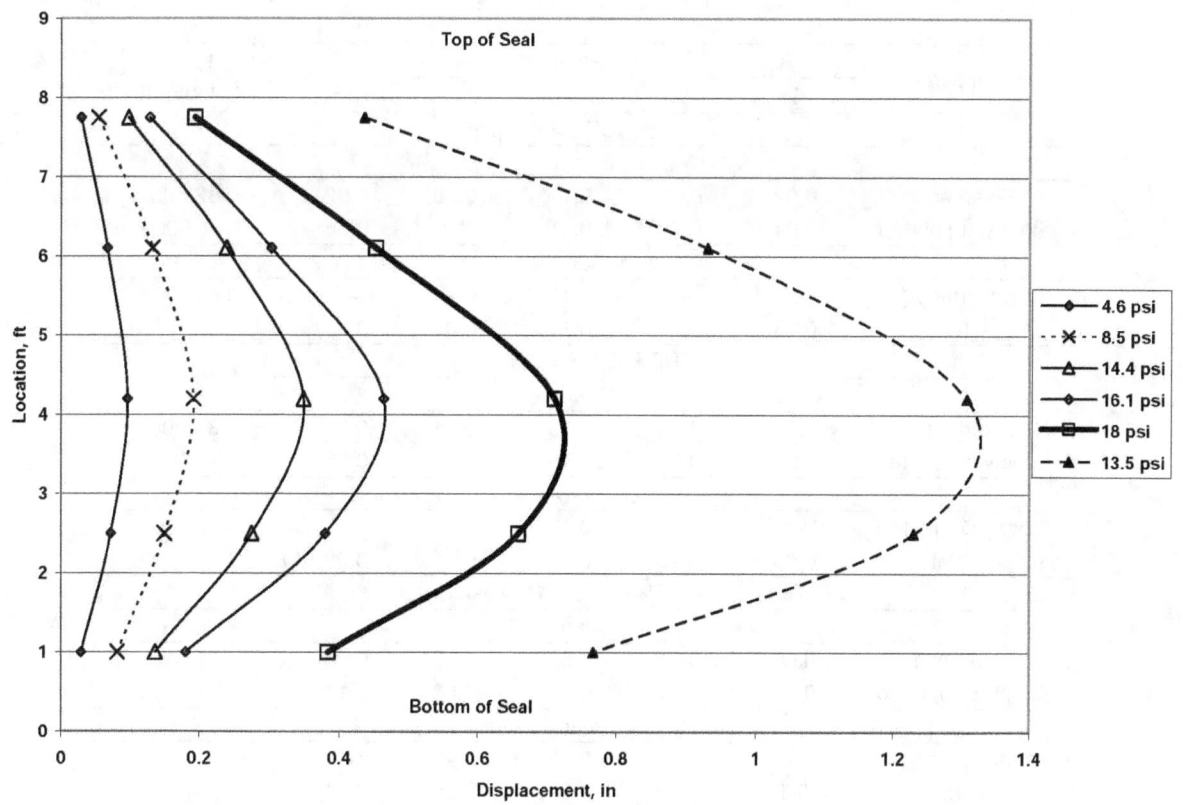

Figure 25.—Displacements along vertical center line of the seal show the change in shape of the seal during the test for a given transducer pressure. Curves to the right of the 18-psi line represent the behavior after the peak pressure was achieved.

Table 5.—Calculated deflections (in inches) of the seal based on assumed end support and the calculated elastic modulus used to match the actual seal deflections at the center of the seal

Support	Location,[1] ft					Elastic modulus, psi
	1	2.5	4.3	6	7.5	
PRESSURE = 4.6 psi						
Beam						
Fixed-end	0.02	0.08	0.11	0.08	0.02	32,500
Simply supported	0.04	0.08	0.11	0.1	0.06	135,000
Plate						
Simply supported	—	—	0.11	—	—	125,000
Actual	0.03	0.08	0.11	0.08	0.03	-
PRESSURE = 8.5 psi						
Beam						
Fixed-end	0.03	0.13	0.19	0.14	0.03	31,000
Simply supported	0.07	0.16	0.19	0.17	0.08	136,000
Plate						
Simply supported	—	—	0.19	—	—	117,000
Actual	0.05	0.13	0.19	0.15	0.08	—
PRESSURE = 14.4 psi						
Beam						
Fixed-end	0.06	0.24	0.35	0.25	0.06	26,500
Simply supported	0.12	0.27	0.35	0.29	0.14	124,000
Plate						
Simply supported	—	—	0.35	—	—	100,000
Actual	0.1	0.24	0.35	0.28	0.14	—
PRESSURE = 16.1 psi						
Beam						
Fixed-end	0.08	0.31	0.46	0.32	0.08	22,500
Simply supported	0.16	0.36	0.46	0.38	0.18	105,000
Plate						
Simply supported	—	—	0.46	—	—	84,000
Actual	0.13	0.3	0.46	0.38	0.18	—

[1]Locations are from the roof.

For the seal, the elastic modulus varies from an average of 828 psi for the polyurethane-aggregate mixture to 6,417 psi for the polyurethane cap. The actual large-scale elastic modulus for the seal is not known, but would not exceed that of the polyurethane cap and would probably be much less. However, using the elastic modulus of the polyurethane cap for the seal, the concrete block walls apparently increase the stiffness of the seal by a factor of 3.5–5.0 for a fixed-end condition and by a factor of 13–19 for a plate with simply supported edges. If the polyurethane-aggregate mixture determines the elastic modulus of the seal, the contribution of the forms to the seal stiffness would be an order of magnitude higher. Therefore, the form walls are substantially increasing the seal stiffness prior to failure. The increased stiffness developed from the block forms prevents the seal core from failing in tension or compression through bending. Therefore, this results in a greater likelihood of a shear failure of the seal to occur. After the seal yields, the form walls offer little resistance to displacement, as indicated by the flattening of the pressure displacement curve (Figure 21). This could imply that the on set of yield may be occurring because of the loss of constraint or support provided by the form walls.

At the lowest pressure, the fixed-end solution is closer to the actual deflections at the points away from the center (see Table 5). At the higher pressures, the simply supported solution generally calculates deflections that are somewhat closer to the measured values. The smooth arc shape of the displacement curves on Figure 25 also indicates that the seal is acting more like a simply supported beam at the higher pressures. This could occur as a result of shearing deformations that may be developing at the ends beyond that due to bending because of the low deformation properties of the seal (Figure 25).

Hydrostatic Versus Explosion Testing of Polyurethane Seals

Explosion testing of polyurethane seals was conducted at the LLEM in the 1990s [Weiss et al. 1996]. These tests were made in openings that were 18 ft wide by 6.5 ft high with an opening area of 120 ft^2. During these tests, the seal thickness, core densities, and types of stacked wall blocks were varied. There were six tests on seals that contained a polyurethane-aggregate mixture; only the results of these tests will be used in the comparison to the seal tested in the hydrostatic chamber. Because of the size difference (both area and thickness) between the seal in the hydrostatic chamber and those in the explosion tests, the shear stresses along the boundaries at failure can be used in comparing the seal performance.

Table 6 summarizes the seal design and shear stresses at failure for the explosion tests. Because the explosion tests are pass/fail, only a range of the possible shear stresses at failure can be determined. All six of the seals are considered to have passed the 20-psi criterion. Four of the seals failed at pressures higher than the criterion, and two seals did not fail during subsequent tests.

Table 6.—Summary of explosion tests on polyurethane-aggregate seals conducted in the 1990s
[Weiss et al. 1996]

Seal No.	Type of block	Designed core thickness, in	Actual core thickness, in	Core density, lb/ft^3	Pressure,[1] psi			Range of possible shear stresses at failure, psi
					Passed	Passed	Failed	
1	HC	30	30	NA	21	NAp	32	20–31
2	HC	18	20	NA	21	39	NAp	>50
3	HC	12	16	NA	21	NAp	40	38–72
8	S	16	16	46	20	28	NAp	>56
9	HC	16	16	40	19	NAp	29	34–52
[2]10	S	18	18	35	19	NAp	24	30–37

HC Hollow core block.   S Solid core block.   NA Not available.   NAp Not applicable.
[1]The seal passed or failed the ventilation test requirements after being subjected to the indicated pressure.
[2]The front form wall contained a pilaster.

Based on these tests, the range of possible shear stresses at failure is 20–72 psi for those seals that were tested to failure. The range of the maximum shear stress possible at failure is 31–72 psi. The maximum possible shear strength is the highest shear strength that could be determined from each test and is calculated from the pressure when the seal failed. The true maximum shear strengths would therefore likely be lower than these values. As previously calculated, the shear stress on the hydrostatically tested seal was 39.4 psi at the maximum pressure. The hydrostatically loaded seal, however, began to yield at a shear stress of 35.3 psi. This places the shear strength of the seal tested in the hydrostatic chamber within the lower range of the maximum shear stresses determined from the explosion tests. The lower strength of the seal may in part be due to the construction flaw on the upper right side of the seal though the seal was in yield.

Further, a direct comparison can be made to the performance of seal 10, the seal most similar in design. The main difference is that seal 10 was constructed with a pilaster in the form wall that could have increased the rigidity of the seal. For seal 10, the possible range of shear stresses at failure is 30–37 psi. Essentially, the shear stresses at failure are nearly the same. This suggests that the two tests can provide similar results and that the shear strengths are relevant to seal design.

However, the conclusions reached from the two types of tests are different. The seals subjected to the explosion tests would be considered to have met the Code of Federal Regulations criterion at the time of the test whereas the hydrostatically loaded seal did not. In part, these seals were designed to meet or exceed the criterion with probably little consideration to a factor of safety. Further, there are too many variables and unknowns involved with this type of seal construction and testing to allow for such precise design and consistent results.

In addition, the seal in the static test may have been subjected to more deformation due to the sustained load than the seal in the explosion test. The increased deformation could lead to the seal fracturing at a lower stress. In part, the time-dependent properties of the polyurethane could cause an increase in the displacement of the seal during the static test, whereas this would not occur during the short period of loading from the explosion tests. Also, a part of the energy during the explosion test is used to accelerate the seal mass and is not available to deform the seal. Therefore, the results of the static test may be more conservative than those of the explosion tests.

For the explosion tests, a minimum seal mass is required to prevent seal failure with the strength of the seals actually increasing with density. However, the effects of the seal mass cannot be evaluated in the static tests. This also suggests that there are other failure criteria related to the dynamic loading that may need to be considered in seal design, and this forms the basis of the minimum density requirements for the seal.

Another difference between the seals tested in the 1990s and the seal tested in the hydrostatic chamber is the uniaxial compressive strength of the polyurethane-aggregate mixture. For the polyurethane aggregate-mixture from the explosion tests, a total of 12 samples were tested in uniaxial compression in the direction perpendicular to foam rise. These samples were obtained from a block of seal material saved from prior testing. These samples had a diameter and length of 6 in and were prepared and tested in the same manner as those from the seal in the hydrostatic chamber. Table 7 shows the average stress at 10% and 30% strain for the 12 samples. These strain levels are used because there is no clear yield or collapse stress for the samples. Also shown in the table is the average stress at 10% and 30% strain for all of the samples tested perpendicular to foam rise for the seal tested in the hydrostatic chamber.

Table 7.—Average strengths of polyurethane-aggregate mixtures tested
perpendicular to foam rise in uniaxial compression
from an explosion-tested seal from the 1990s
and the seal tested in the hydrostatic chamber

No. of samples	Density, lb/ft^3	SD, lb/ft^3	Stress at 10% strain, psi	SD, psi	Stress at 30% strain, psi	SD, psi
SEAL TESTED IN HYDROSTATIC CHAMBER						
13	33.7	4.8	31.7	6.9	85	24
EXPLOSION-TESTED SEAL, 1990s						
12	40.6	3.1	59	14	188	26

SD   Standard deviation.

Figure 26 shows some stress-strain curves for samples tested in compression for the poly-urethane cap and polyurethane-aggregate mixture from the explosion-tested seal and the seal tested in the hydrostatic chamber. All three samples were tested in the direction perpendicular to foam rise. The densities of the samples were 11 lb/ft^3 for the polyurethane cap, 46 lb/ft^3 for the polyurethane-aggregate mixture from the explosion-tested seal, and 31 lb/ft^3 for the polyurethane-aggregate mixture from the hydrostatically tested seal.

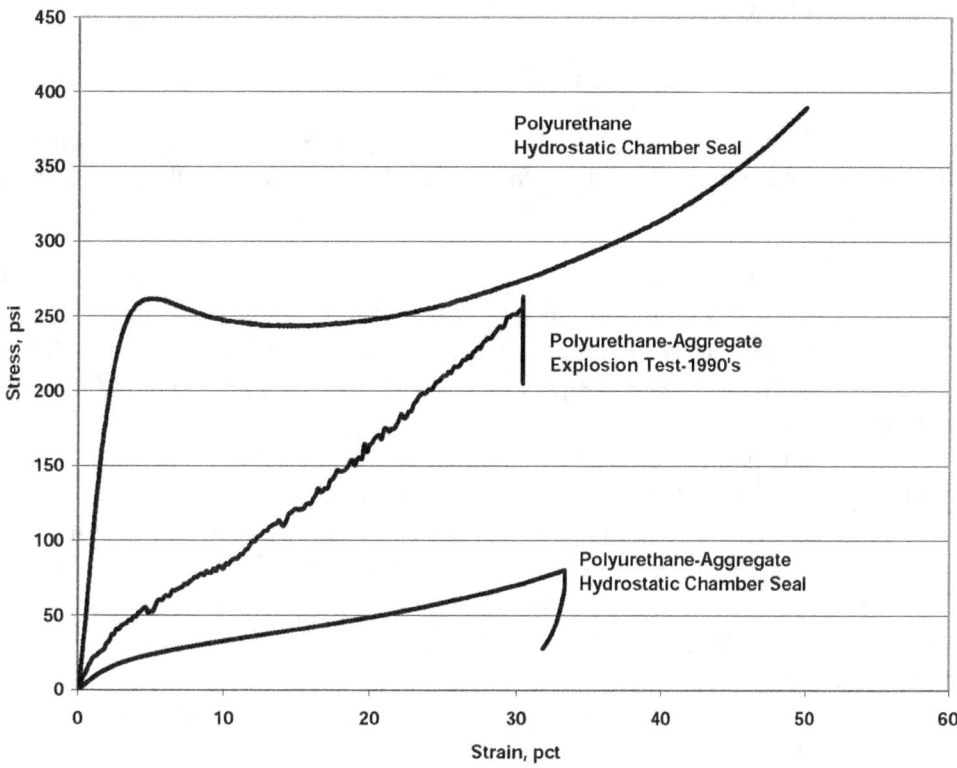

Figure 26.—Stress-strain curves from uniaxial compressive tests on samples from explosion-tested seal from the 1990s and the seal tested in the hydrostatic chamber. Direction of testing was perpendicular to foam rise. The samples were either pure polyurethane or a polyurethane-aggregate mixture.

The compressive test results indicate that the strength and stiffness of the polyurethane-aggregate mixture from both sets of seals were degraded significantly from those of the polyurethane only. However, the polyurethane-aggregate mixture from the explosion-tested seal from the 1990s showed much less decrease in strength and stiffness. The polyurethane aggregate from the 1990s seal has about twice the strength at 10% and 30% strain compared to the polyurethane-aggregate mixture from the more recent hydrostatically tested seal. The degradation of the strength of the polyurethane-aggregate mixture of the explosion-tested seal resulted from the formation of a small amount of soft foam around each aggregate similar to that occurring in the polyurethane-aggregate mixture from the seal tested in the hydrostatic chamber.

Essentially, moisture seems to reduce the strength of the polyurethane-aggregate mixture for both the seal tested in the hydrostatic chamber and the explosion-tested seal from the 1990s by causing the formation of soft foam around the aggregate. Apparently, however, the polyurethane-aggregate mixture from the explosion-tested seal was affected to a lesser degree. Because the compressive strength is much less for the polyurethane-aggregate mixture from the more recent seal tested in the hydrostatic chamber, the results of the explosion tests conducted in the 1990s may not be applicable for establishing design criteria for seals constructed today. Since the seal tested in the hydrostatic chamber did not meet the 20-psi criterion either because of the reduced strength or the construction flaw, there seems to be at present no solid technical basis to establish the minimum design requirement for such seals from the results of full-scale physical testing. Unless the amount of the soft foam and construction flaws can be controlled or eliminated, significant safety factors will need to be used in the design of seals built with a polyurethane-aggregate mixture.

CONCLUSIONS

From the test of the composite polyurethane-aggregate seal in the hydrostatic chamber and the results of the testing of the seal material, several conclusions about the seal performance can be reached.

1. The average pressure applied to the seal at failure was 18.9 psi. This is less than the 20 psi of horizontal static pressure established in the Code of Federal Regulations (at the time of the test) for such a seal [30 CFR 75 (2005)]. Therefore, this seal did not meet the regulatory requirements when the horizontal static pressure was applied with water.
2. The seal yielded structurally at an average hydraulic pressure of 17 psi. This was accompanied by increased damage and water leakage.
3. Based on the observed damage to the seal and the measured displacements, the failure initiated from shear near the top and along the right side of the seal. This occurred along a construction flaw, a zone with a high aggregate content but poorly bonded with the polyurethane. The seal then failed along the lower center and left side of the seal.
4. The addition of the aggregate altered the characteristics and properties of the foam in the polyurethane-aggregate mixture. A high percentage of the foam in the polyurethane-aggregate mixture developed into a soft foam that can carry little load prior to the collapse of the foam structure. Further, the density of the foam in the mixture is less than half of that for the polyurethane cap and less than the minimum design density. These changes have resulted in large reductions in the strength and stiffness of the polyurethane-aggregate mixture compared to the polyurethane foam

with no aggregate. Further, the reduction in foam density in the mixture resulted in the overall seal density being less than the minimum required to resist the energy of an explosion.

5. The change in foam characteristics in the mixture seems to be caused by moisture associated with the aggregate. Steps were taken to minimize the effects of the moisture, but were not successful.

6. The change in characteristics and properties of the foam in the mixture is important because the polyurethane-aggregate mixture comprises at least 80% by volume of the seal. Further, it seems that the failures have occurred through the polyurethane-aggregate mixture in the seal. Therefore, the change in foam characteristics as a result of the addition of the aggregate has reduced the overall stiffness and strength of the seal.

7. The calculated shear stresses at failure and the estimated shear strength of the polyurethane-aggregate mixture are fairly close. This suggests that the strength and properties of the polyurethane-aggregate mixture controlled the maximum static pressure that the seal could withstand.

8. The concrete block form walls added considerable stiffness to the seal, which minimizes the amount of prefailure deflection. This composite behavior may reduce the potential for a tension or compression failure in bending resulting in the seal failing in shear.

9. Polyurethane-aggregate seals constructed and tested in the 1990s passed the 20-psi criterion, but the recently tested seal in the hydrostatic chamber did not. The difference in the outcomes seems to be related to a difference in the strength and stiffness properties between the seals. Therefore, it is questionable whether the results of the seals tested in the 1990s should be used in establishing or confirming the design criteria for these types of seals. Since, the polyurethane-aggregate seal tested in the hydrostatic chamber did not meet the criteria, there are then no results from full-scale physical testing that can be used to establish or confirm minimum design requirements for such seals.

10. Because the formation of the soft foam seems to be highly variable and may be difficult to control, significant safety factors need to be built into the design of the seals using a polyurethane-aggregate mixture. To reduce the formation of soft foam, techniques could be developed to control the moisture.

11. The joints between the lifts are weaker in tension than the surrounding polyurethane or polyurethane-aggregate mixture. Further, other defects in the form of long narrow fissures in the polyurethane cap developed in the seal. Although the joints and fissures have the potential to decrease the seal strength, these features do not seem to have contributed to the seal failure in this case.

REFERENCES

72 Fed. Reg. 28795 [2007]. Mine Safety and Health Administration: sealing of abandoned areas; final rule (30 CFR part 75).

ASTM [2004a]. Standard test method for apparent density of rigid cellular plastics. West Conshohocken, PA: ASTM International. ASTM D1622–03.

ASTM [2004b]. Standard test method for compressive properties of rigid cellular plastics. West Conshohocken, PA: ASTM International. ASTM D1621–04a.

ASTM [2004c]. Standard test methods for density and specific gravity (relative density) of plastics by displacement. West Conshohocken, PA: ASTM International. ASTM D792–00.

CFR. Code of Federal regulations. Washington, DC: U.S. Government Printing Office, Office of the Federal Register.

DuPont [1987]. Freon product information. Properties of rigid urethane foams. Bulletin BA–13. Wilmington, DE: E. I. DuPont de Nemours & Co, Inc.

Hawkins MC, O'Toole B, Jackovich D [2005]. Cell morphology and mechanical properties of rigid polyurethane foam. J Cell Plastics *41*(3):267–285.

Huber AT, Gibson LJ [1988]. Anisotropy of foams. J Mater Sci *23*(8):3031–3040.

MSHA [1996]. Report of investigation (underground coal mine). Noninjury coal mine explosion. Mine No. 1 (I.D. No. 46–07273), Oasis Contracting, Inc., Quinland, Boone County, West Virginia, May 15, 1996, and June 22, 1996. U.S. Department of Labor, Mine Safety and Health Administration.

Obert L, Duvall WI [1967]. Rock mechanics and the design of structures in rock. New York: John Wiley and Sons.

Piping Technology & Products [2008]. Polyurethane technical information. [http://www.pipingtech.com/products/preis/poly.pdf]. Date accessed: February 2008.

Sapko MJ, Weiss ES [2001]. Evaluation of new methods and facilities to test explosion-resistant seals. In: Proceedings of the 29th International Conference of Safety in Mines Research Institutes (October 8–11, 2001). Vol. 1. Katowice, Poland: Central Mining Institute, pp. 157–166.

Sapko MJ, Weiss ES, Cashdollar KL, Greninger NB [1999a]. Overview of NIOSH's mine seal research. In: Proceedings of the 28th International Conference of Safety in Mines Research Institutes (Sinaia, Romania). Vol. I, pp. 71–85.

Sapko MJ, Weiss ES, Greninger NB [1999b]. Recent mine seal research conducted by NIOSH. In: Sealbarr '99 - Proceedings of the Polish-American Seminar on Seals and Barriers as a Means of Protection Against Fires and Explosions in Mines (Katowice, Poland, May 27–28, 1999), pp. 39–53.

Sapko MJ, Weiss ES, Harteis SP [2003]. Alternative methodologies for evaluating explosion-resistant mine ventilation seals. In: Proceedings of the 30th International Conference of Safety in Mines Research Institutes. Johannesburg, Republic of South Africa: South African Institute of Mining and Metallurgy, pp. 615–640.

Sawyer SG Jr. [1999]. A computational analysis method to determine the thickness required for polyurethane/limestone mine seals in large openings [Thesis]. Pittsburgh, PA: Carnegie Mellon University, Department of Civil and Environmental Engineering.

Triebsch G, Sapko MJ [1990]. Lake Lynn Laboratory: a state-of-the-art mining research laboratory. In: Proceedings of the International Symposium on Unique Underground Structures. Vol. 2. Golden, CO: Colorado School of Mines, pp. 75–1 to 75–21.

Weiss ES, Slivensky WA, Schultz MJ, Stephan CR. Jackson KW [1996]. Evaluation of polymer construction material and water trap designs for underground coal mine seals. Pittsburgh, PA: U.S. Department of Energy, RI 9634. NTIS No. PB96–123392.

Zhang J (JYZQA@claytoncorp.com) [2006]. Comments on polyurethane foam. E-mail message to Michael J. Sapko (NIOSH Pittsburgh Research Laboratory), March 17.

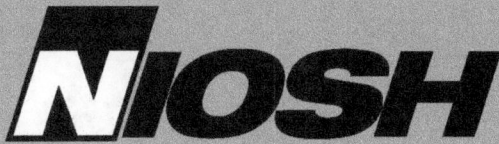

Delivering on the Nation's promise:
safety and health at work for all people
through research and prevention

To receive NIOSH documents or more information about
occupational safety and health topics, contact NIOSH at

1–800–CDC–INFO (1–800–232–4636)
TTY: 1–888–232–6348
e-mail: cdcinfo@cdc.gov

or visit the NIOSH Web site at **www.cdc.gov/niosh.**

For a monthly update on news at NIOSH, subscribe to
NIOSH *eNews* by visiting **www.cdc.gov/niosh/eNews.**

DHHS (NIOSH) Publication No. 2008–129

SAFER • HEALTHIER • PEOPLE™

www.ingramcontent.com/pod-product-compliance
Lightning Source LLC
Chambersburg PA
CBHW080923290526
45795CB00007BA/2628